Vivienne Beaufoy

The Key To Proper Nutrition and Weight Management

This book was professionally typeset on Reedsy

Find out more at reedsy.com

Contents

1.

2.

3.

4.

5.

6.

7.

8.

9.

10.

11.

12.

13.

14.

15.

16.

17.

18.

19.

20.

21.

22.

23.

24.

25.

26.

27.

28.

29.

30.

31.

32.

33.

34.

35.

36.

37.

38.

39.

40.

41.

42.

43.

44.

45.

46.

47.

48.

49.

50.

51.

Chapter 1: Understanding the Fundamentals of Nutrition

1.1 Introduction to Nutrition

Nutrition is the science of how the body utilizes nutrients from the foods we consume to support growth, development, and overall health. It plays a pivotal role in maintaining bodily functions, providing energy, and preventing various diseases. Proper nutrition involves the consumption of a balanced diet that contains essential nutrients in adequate proportions. By understanding nutrition, individuals can make informed food choices to promote well-being and achieve their health goals.

Nutrition encompasses a wide range of topics, including macronutrients (carbohydrates, proteins, and fats), micronutrients (vitamins and minerals), and the significance of various foods in our diets. A healthy and balanced diet provides the necessary nutrients to maintain optimal health, support immune function, and prevent chronic conditions such as obesity, diabetes, and cardiovascular diseases.

1.2 Nutrients: Macro and Micronutrients

Nutrients are substances that the body requires for growth, energy, and proper functioning. They can be categorized into two main groups: macronutrients and micronutrients.

Macronutrients are nutrients that the body needs in large quantities. They include carbohydrates, proteins, and fats. Carbohydrates are the primary source of energy and are found in foods like grains, fruits, and vegetables. Proteins are essential for tissue repair, muscle growth, and hormone synthesis, and they are present in foods such as meat, legumes, and dairy products. Fats are critical for energy storage, cell structure, and hormone production, and they can be found in oils, nuts, and avocados.

Micronutrients are nutrients that the body requires in smaller amounts, but they are equally vital for various physiological processes. These include vitamins (e.g., vitamin A, vitamin C) and minerals (e.g., calcium, iron, zinc). Micronutrients play crucial roles in immune function, bone health, metabolism, and antioxidant defense.

1.3 The Importance of a Balanced Diet

A balanced diet is one that provides all the essential nutrients in appropriate proportions to meet the body's needs. Consuming a wide variety of foods from different food groups ensures that individuals get the necessary nutrients for overall health. A balanced diet is essential for maintaining a healthy weight, promoting proper growth and development, and reducing the risk of chronic diseases.

A balanced diet should include a mix of whole grains, lean proteins, healthy fats, fruits, and vegetables. It should limit the intake of added sugars, sodium, and unhealthy fats. By following a balanced diet, individuals can achieve and maintain a healthy body composition, support immune function, and improve overall well-being.

1.4 Digestion and Absorption

Digestion is the process by which the body breaks down food into smaller molecules that can be absorbed and utilized. It begins in the mouth, where enzymes start breaking down carbohydrates through chewing and salivary amylase. The partially digested food then travels to the stomach, where gastric juices aid in further breakdown of proteins.

From the stomach, the food moves into the small intestine, where most digestion and nutrient absorption take place. Here, enzymes from the pancreas and bile from the liver break down fats, proteins, and carbohydrates into their constituent parts. Nutrients are then absorbed through the intestinal lining and transported to various body tissues via the bloodstream.

The large intestine is responsible for absorbing water and electrolytes, while also playing a role in fermenting certain fibers by gut bacteria. Finally, waste products are eliminated from the body through bowel movements.

1.5 Nutritional Guidelines and Recommendations

Nutritional guidelines and recommendations are set by health authorities and organizations to guide individuals in making healthy food choices. These guidelines are based on scientific research and aim to promote overall health and prevent diet-related diseases.

In the United States, the Dietary Guidelines for Americans, published every five years by the U.S. Department of Agriculture (USDA) and the U.S. Department of Health and Human Services (HHS), provide evidence-based recommendations for individuals aged 2 and older. The guidelines emphasize the consumption of nutrient-dense foods, such as fruits, vegetables, whole grains, lean proteins, and low-fat dairy products, while limiting added sugars, sodium, and saturated fats.

Other countries and international organizations, such as the World Health Organization (WHO) and the Food and Agriculture Organization (FAO) of the United Nations, also issue their own dietary guidelines and recommendations tailored to their populations.

1.6 The Role of Nutraceuticals and Functional Foods

Nutraceuticals are products derived from food sources with potential health benefits beyond basic nutrition. They may offer protective effects against certain diseases or support overall well-being. Examples of nutraceuticals include omega-3 fatty acids, probiotics, and plant-based extracts like green tea polyphenols.

Functional foods are foods or food components that provide specific health benefits beyond their basic nutritional value. They are typically enriched with bioactive compounds or nutrients to promote health. For instance, fortified milk with added vitamin D for bone health or yogurt with probiotics for gut health are examples of functional foods.

Consuming nutraceuticals and functional foods can be a convenient way to obtain specific health benefits, but it is essential to consult with healthcare professionals before incorporating them into one's diet, especially if there are existing health conditions or medications involved.

1.7 Nutritional Myths and Misconceptions

Nutrition is a subject that is often surrounded by myths and misconceptions. These misinformation can lead to confusion and poor dietary choices. Some common nutritional myths include:

- Myth: Carbohydrates are inherently fattening and should be avoided for weight loss.
   - Myth: Fat-free or low-fat foods are always healthier than their full-fat counterparts.
   - Myth: Consuming certain foods can "burn fat" or lead to spot reduction of body fat.
   - Myth: Skipping meals is an effective way to lose weight.
   - Myth: All processed foods are unhealthy and should be avoided entirely.

To make informed decisions about nutrition, it is crucial to rely on evidence-based information from reputable sources, such as registered dietitians, nutritionists, and authoritative health organizations.

1.8 Maintaining a Healthy Relationship with Food

Developing a healthy relationship with food is essential for overall well-being and balanced eating habits. A positive relationship with food involves recognizing hunger and fullness cues, enjoying a wide variety of foods, and avoiding restrictive or obsessive eating patterns.

Practicing mindful eating, which involves being present and fully engaged while eating, can help improve the relationship with food. By paying attention to hunger and satiety signals, individuals can better regulate their food intake and avoid overeating or emotional eating.

It is crucial to embrace food as a source of nourishment and pleasure rather than a source of guilt or punishment. Allowing occasional indulgences in favorite foods can be part of a healthy relationship with food, as long as it is balanced with overall nutrient-dense choices.

1.9 Building Sustainable Eating Habits

Sustainability in nutrition refers to adopting dietary habits that are both health-promoting and environmentally friendly. Building sustainable eating habits involves considering the impact of food choices on personal health and the planet.

To promote sustainability, individuals can:

- Choose plant-based options more often: Plant-based diets are associated with lower environmental footprints and can be nutritious when well-planned.

- Reduce food waste: Plan meals, use leftovers, and compost food scraps to minimize waste.

- Support local and seasonal produce: Buying locally grown and seasonal foods reduces the carbon footprint associated with transportation.

- Opt for sustainably sourced seafood: Choose

seafood that is caught or farmed using methods that protect marine ecosystems and species.

By making conscious choices and embracing sustainable eating habits, individuals can contribute to their own health and the health of the planet.

1.10 Tracking and Assessing Your Nutritional Intake

Keeping track of nutritional intake can help individuals gain insight into their dietary habits and make necessary adjustments. Various tools and methods are available for tracking nutrition, including food diaries, mobile apps, and online nutrient databases.

Food diaries involve writing down everything consumed throughout the day, including portion sizes. Mobile apps and online databases can simplify the process by providing nutrient information for thousands of foods.

Nutritional assessments can also be conducted by healthcare professionals, such as registered dietitians, to evaluate dietary patterns and identify potential nutrient deficiencies or excesses. These assessments consider factors such as age, sex, activity level, and health goals.

Tracking and assessing nutritional intake can be especially beneficial for individuals with specific health conditions or those working towards weight management goals. It empowers individuals to make informed decisions about their diets and work towards a healthier lifestyle.

Chapter 2: Protein - The Building Block of Life

2.1 Understanding Protein and Amino Acids

Protein is an essential macronutrient that plays a critical role in the structure, function, and regulation of the body's cells and tissues. It is made up of smaller units called amino acids, which are linked together in specific sequences. There are 20 different amino acids that combine to form proteins, and they are classified into essential and non-essential amino acids.

Essential amino acids are those that the body cannot produce on its own and must be obtained through the diet. Non-essential amino acids, on the other hand, can be synthesized by the body. Both types of amino acids are vital for various physiological processes, such as building and repairing tissues, supporting the immune system, and producing enzymes and hormones.

2.2 Complete vs. Incomplete Proteins

Proteins from different sources can be classified as complete or incomplete based on their amino acid profile. Complete proteins contain all nine essential amino acids in sufficient quantities to meet the body's needs. Animal-based protein sources, such as meat, fish, eggs, and dairy, are generally complete proteins.

Incomplete proteins lack one or more essential amino acids or have inadequate amounts of them. Most plant-based protein sources, such as legumes, grains, nuts, and seeds, fall into this category. However, by combining various plant-based protein sources, individuals can create complementary proteins that provide all essential amino acids. For example, combining rice and beans or whole-grain bread with peanut butter can form a complete protein.

2.3 Protein's Role in Muscle Building and Repair

Protein is essential for muscle building, repair, and maintenance. During physical activity or resistance training, muscle fibers experience microscopic damage. Protein-rich diets support the repair and growth of these muscles, leading to increased strength and muscle mass.

Muscles are composed mainly of two proteins: actin and myosin. The body breaks down dietary proteins into amino acids during digestion. These amino acids are then used to synthesize new proteins, which are incorporated into muscle fibers during the repair and growth process.

Athletes, bodybuilders, and individuals engaging in regular physical activity often have increased protein needs to support muscle repair and development. Proper protein intake, combined with an appropriate exercise regimen, is essential for achieving fitness goals and maintaining overall health.

2.4 Plant-Based Protein Sources

Plant-based protein sources offer an array of nutrients while contributing to a sustainable and environmentally friendly diet. They are rich in fiber, vitamins, minerals, and phytonutrients that promote overall health. Some common plant-based protein sources include:

- Legumes: Beans, lentils, chickpeas, and peas are excellent sources of protein and also provide complex carbohydrates and fiber.
- Grains: Whole grains like quinoa, brown rice, and oats contain protein along with essential nutrients and dietary fiber.
- Nuts and Seeds: Almonds, walnuts, chia seeds, and hemp seeds are protein-rich and also supply healthy fats and micronutrients.
- Soy: Soy products, such as tofu, tempeh, and edamame, are complete sources of plant-based protein.

Plant-based diets can provide adequate protein when a variety of protein sources are included and complemented to ensure a balance of essential amino acids.

2.5 Animal-Based Protein Sources

Animal-based protein sources are considered complete proteins as they contain all essential amino acids in sufficient quantities. They are particularly rich in high-quality proteins that are easily digestible and readily available for the body's needs. Some common animal-based protein sources include:

- Meat: Beef, poultry, pork, and lamb are rich in protein, iron, zinc, and B-vitamins.

- Fish and Seafood: Fish such as salmon, tuna, and trout provide protein along with omega-3 fatty acids, which are beneficial for heart health.

- Eggs: Eggs are a complete protein source and also contain essential nutrients like vitamin B12 and choline.

- Dairy: Milk, yogurt, and cheese are excellent sources of protein and calcium, important for bone health.

Animal-based proteins can be incorporated into a balanced diet, but it is essential to be mindful of the overall dietary pattern and consider factors like saturated fat and cholesterol content.

2.6 Protein Quality and Bioavailability

Protein quality refers to how well a protein source provides essential amino acids and supports the body's protein needs. Factors such as the amino acid composition, digestibility, and bioavailability determine protein quality.

Animal-based proteins are generally considered high-quality proteins due to their complete amino acid profile and high digestibility. Plant-based proteins may vary in quality, with some being incomplete or less digestible than animal-based sources.

The concept of protein bioavailability relates to the proportion of ingested protein that the body can absorb and utilize. Animal-based proteins often have higher bioavailability compared to plant-based proteins. However, by combining different plant-based protein sources and consuming a varied diet, individuals can enhance the overall bioavailability of plant-based proteins.

2.7 Protein Requirements for Different Lifestages

Protein requirements vary depending on factors such as age, sex, activity level, and overall health. During different lifestages, protein needs may change to support growth, development, and other physiological changes. The Recommended Dietary Allowance (RDA) for protein is set by health authorities based on age and sex:

- Infants (0-6 months): 9.1 grams/day
    - Infants (7-12 months): 11 grams/day
    - Children (1-3 years): 13 grams/day
    - Children (4-8 years): 19 grams/day
    - Boys (9-13 years): 34 grams/day
    - Boys (14-18 years): 52 grams/day
    - Girls (9-13 years): 34 grams/day
    - Girls (14-18 years): 46 grams/day

For adults, the RDA for protein is approximately 0.8 grams of protein per kilogram of body weight per day. However, individual protein needs may vary based on factors like physical activity, muscle mass, and overall health goals.

Pregnant and breastfeeding women require additional protein to support fetal and infant growth and development. Athletes and individuals engaged in intense physical activity may also need more protein to support muscle repair and recovery.

It is essential to consult with healthcare professionals or registered dietitians to determine individualized protein needs and ensure adequate intake at different lifestages.

2.8 Combining Proteins for Optimal Nutrition

For individuals following plant-based diets or those looking to diversify their protein sources, combining complementary proteins can be an effective strategy to ensure adequate intake of essential amino acids. Complementary proteins are two or more protein sources that, when combined, provide all the essential amino acids in sufficient quantities.

Examples of complementary protein combinations include:

- Rice and beans: This classic combination provides all essential amino acids.

- Whole-grain bread with peanut butter: The combination of grains and nuts supplies complete protein.

- Lentils with whole grains: Lentils and whole grains like quinoa or brown rice complement each other to form complete protein.

By incorporating a variety of plant-based protein sources and pairing them strategically, individuals can achieve a balanced and complete protein intake.

2.9 Debunking Protein Myths

Protein has been the subject of various myths and misconceptions. It is essential to address these myths to make informed decisions about dietary choices. Some common protein myths include:

- Myth: High protein diets are harmful to kidney function. Truth: High protein intake

may be a concern for individuals with pre-existing kidney conditions, but for healthy individuals, moderate protein intake is safe.

- Myth: Protein supplements are necessary for muscle gain. Truth: While protein supplements can be convenient, whole food sources can provide adequate protein for muscle building and repair.

- Myth: Animal-based proteins are superior to plant-based proteins. Truth: Both animal and plant-based proteins can contribute to a healthy diet when chosen wisely and in combination to meet essential amino acid requirements.

- Myth: Eating too much protein can lead to weight gain. Truth: Weight gain is determined by overall caloric intake and energy balance. Protein can support satiety and muscle preservation during weight loss.

It is essential to rely on evidence-based information and consult with healthcare professionals for personalized dietary advice.

2.10 Protein Supplementation and Safety

Protein supplementation, such as protein powders and shakes, is a popular option for individuals seeking convenient ways to increase protein intake or support fitness goals. Protein supplements can be beneficial for athletes, individuals with increased protein needs, or those with limited access to whole food protein sources.

When choosing protein supplements, it is essential to consider factors such as protein quality, ingredient list, and potential allergens. Some protein supplements are derived from dairy (whey or casein), while others come from plant-based sources (soy, pea, hemp). It is crucial to choose products that align with dietary preferences and restrictions.

While protein supplementation can be safe for many individuals, excessive use may lead to an imbalance of nutrients or excessive calorie intake. Additionally, some protein supplements may contain added sugars, artificial flavors, or other additives, which should be considered when selecting products.

As with any dietary supplement, it is advisable to consult with healthcare professionals or registered dietitians before starting protein supplementation, especially for those with pre-existing health conditions or specific dietary needs.

In conclusion, protein is a fundamental macronutrient that serves as the building block of life. Understanding the role of protein and amino acids, different sources of proteins, and their bioavailability is essential for meeting individual nutritional needs. Whether from animal-based or plant-based sources, protein can be a part of a balanced and nutritious diet. By incorporating a variety of protein sources and practicing mindful eating, individuals can achieve optimal nutrition and support their overall health and wellness.

Chapter 3: Smart Carbohydrates for Energy and Vitality

3.1 Understanding Carbohydrates: Sugars, Starches, and Fiber

Carbohydrates are one of the three main macronutrients, along with proteins and fats, that provide energy for the body. They are composed of carbon, hydrogen, and oxygen molecules and can be classified into three main types: sugars, starches, and fiber.

Sugars are simple carbohydrates that consist of one or two sugar molecules. They are found naturally in foods like fruits (fructose) and milk (lactose), as well as in added sugars present in processed foods and sweetened beverages. While some natural sugars come with beneficial nutrients and fiber, added sugars provide empty calories and can contribute to weight gain and other health issues.

Starches are complex carbohydrates made up of multiple sugar molecules bonded together. They are the primary form of energy storage in plants and are found in foods such as grains (wheat, rice, oats), legumes (beans, lentils), and starchy vegetables (potatoes, corn).

Fiber is another type of complex carbohydrate that the human body cannot digest. It is found in plant-based foods like fruits, vegetables, whole grains, nuts, and seeds. Fiber provides various health benefits, including promoting digestive health, supporting weight management, and reducing the risk of heart disease.

3.2 The Glycemic Index and Glycemic Load

The glycemic index (GI) is a scale that ranks carbohydrates based on their effect on blood sugar levels. Carbohydrates with a high GI are rapidly digested and cause a quick and significant rise in blood sugar, while those with a low GI are digested more slowly, leading to a gradual increase in blood sugar.

Foods with a high GI include white bread, white rice, and sugary snacks. On the other hand, foods with a low GI include whole grains, legumes, and most fruits and vegetables. Including low-GI foods in the diet can help stabilize blood sugar levels, provide sustained energy, and reduce the risk of type 2 diabetes and cardiovascular disease.

The glycemic load (GL) takes into account both the GI and the amount of carbohydrates in a food. It provides a more accurate picture of how a food affects blood sugar levels. Foods with a high GL have a more significant impact on blood sugar levels compared to foods with a low GL.

Balancing the intake of high-GI foods with low-GI options can help regulate blood sugar levels and support overall health.

3.3 Simple vs. Complex Carbohydrates

Carbohydrates can be further categorized as simple or complex based on their chemical structure and how quickly they are digested.

Simple carbohydrates consist of one or two sugar molecules and are quickly absorbed into the bloodstream, leading to a rapid increase in blood sugar levels. These carbohydrates are found in sugary foods, such as candies, soda, and baked goods. While they can provide a quick source of energy, excessive consumption of simple carbohydrates can lead to fluctuations in blood sugar levels and contribute to weight gain.

Complex carbohydrates, as mentioned earlier, are made up of multiple sugar molecules bonded together. They take longer to break down and provide a steady release of energy over time. Foods rich in complex carbohydrates include whole grains, vegetables, legumes, and fruits. These foods are also typically higher in fiber, vitamins, minerals, and other beneficial nutrients, making them a more nutritious choice compared to simple carbohydrates.

Choosing complex carbohydrates over simple carbohydrates is recommended for stable energy levels, better nutrient intake, and overall health.

3.4 Carbohydrates and Blood Sugar Regulation

Carbohydrates play a significant role in blood sugar regulation. When we consume carbohydrates, they are broken down into glucose, the primary source of energy for the body's cells. Insulin, a hormone produced by the pancreas, helps regulate blood sugar levels by facilitating the uptake of glucose into cells.

Consuming carbohydrates with a high glycemic index can lead to rapid spikes in blood sugar levels, causing a corresponding surge in insulin production. Over time, frequent and sharp fluctuations in blood sugar and insulin levels can contribute to insulin resistance, a condition in which cells become less responsive to insulin. This can lead to the development of type 2 diabetes and other metabolic disorders.

On the other hand, consuming carbohydrates with a low glycemic index promotes more stable blood sugar levels and reduces the demand for insulin. This can help prevent insulin resistance and support overall metabolic health.

Balancing carbohydrate intake, choosing low-GI options, and pairing carbohydrates with proteins and healthy fats can help regulate blood sugar levels and support insulin sensitivity.

3.5 Whole Grains and Their Health Benefits

Whole grains are an essential source of complex carbohydrates that offer a wide array of health benefits. Unlike refined grains, such as white rice and white bread, whole grains retain all parts of the grain kernel—the bran, germ, and endosperm—providing more fiber, vitamins, minerals, and phytonutrients.

The fiber in whole grains supports digestive health by promoting regular bowel movements and reducing the risk of constipation and diverticular disease. It also helps regulate blood sugar levels and supports heart health by lowering LDL cholesterol levels.

Whole grains are rich in B-vitamins, which play essential roles in energy metabolism and nervous system function. Additionally, they provide valuable minerals like iron, magnesium, and zinc, which are necessary for various physiological processes.

Incorporating a variety of whole grains into the diet, such as oats, quinoa, brown rice, and whole wheat, can contribute to better nutrient intake and improved overall health.

3.6 Fruits and Vegetables as Nutrient-Dense Carbohydrate Sources

Fruits and vegetables are nutrient-dense carbohydrate sources that provide an abundance of vitamins, minerals, fiber, and antioxidants. They are essential components of a balanced diet and offer various health benefits.

Fruits are rich in vitamins C and A, potassium, folate, and dietary fiber. They provide natural sweetness while contributing to overall hydration and digestive health. The wide range of phytonutrients in fruits has been associated with a reduced risk of chronic diseases, including heart disease and certain cancers.

Vegetables are packed with vitamins A, C, and K, as well as potassium, magnesium, and dietary fiber. They are low in calories and high in nutrients, making them an excellent choice for weight management and overall health. The antioxidants found in vegetables can neutralize harmful free radicals in the body and protect against oxidative stress and inflammation.

By incorporating a colorful variety of fruits and vegetables into the diet, individuals can enhance their nutrient intake and support their immune system and overall well-being.

3.7 Carbohydrate Timing for Athletes and Active Individuals

For athletes and individuals engaged in regular physical activity, timing carbohydrate intake can significantly impact performance and recovery.

Before exercise: Consuming carbohydrates before exercise can provide a readily available source of energy and support optimal performance. Choosing carbohydrates with a moderate to low glycemic index can provide sustained energy without causing blood sugar spikes.

During exercise: During prolonged or intense exercise, consuming carbohydrates can help maintain energy levels and delay fatigue. Sports drinks, gels, or easily digestible carbohydrates like bananas or energy bars can be effective options.

After exercise: Post-exercise, consuming carbohydrates, along with protein, is crucial for replenishing glycogen stores and promoting muscle recovery. Whole foods like fruits, whole grains, and lean proteins are excellent choices for post-workout meals or snacks.

The timing and amount of carbohydrates required may vary depending on the type, duration, and intensity of

the physical activity, as well as individual training goals and preferences.

3.8 Carbohydrate Intolerance and Management

Some individuals may have carbohydrate intolerance, which refers to difficulty digesting or processing certain carbohydrates. Common examples include lactose intolerance (difficulty digesting lactose in dairy products) and fructose malabsorption (difficulty absorbing fructose in fruits).

For individuals with carbohydrate intolerance, managing their carbohydrate intake and choosing alternatives may be necessary to prevent digestive discomfort and other symptoms. Lactose-free dairy products and low-fructose fruits are examples of suitable alternatives.

Additionally, some individuals may follow low-carbohydrate diets for specific health conditions, such as diabetes or metabolic syndrome. These diets aim to regulate blood sugar levels and improve insulin sensitivity. In such cases, it is essential to work with healthcare professionals or registered dietitians to ensure adequate nutrient intake and balanced dietary choices.

3.9 Balancing Carbohydrates with Other Nutrients

Carbohydrates are a crucial component of a balanced diet, but they should be balanced with other nutrients to support overall health. Protein and healthy fats, for example, are essential for satiety, hormone regulation, and various physiological processes.

Pairing carbohydrates with protein and healthy fats can slow down the absorption of glucose, leading to more stable blood sugar levels and sustained energy. For instance, a balanced meal could include grilled chicken with a side of quinoa and roasted vegetables or a smoothie made with fruit, Greek yogurt, and almond butter.

Choosing nutrient-dense carbohydrates, such as whole grains, fruits, and vegetables, along with a variety of protein sources and healthy fats, can help individuals maintain a balanced and nourishing diet.

3.10 The Role of Carbohydrates in Weight Management

Carbohydrates can play a significant role in weight management when chosen wisely and consumed in appropriate portions.

Fiber-rich carbohydrates, such as whole grains, fruits, and vegetables, promote satiety and help individuals feel fuller for longer. This can aid in reducing overall calorie intake and supporting weight loss or weight maintenance goals.

It is essential to be mindful of portion sizes and avoid excessive consumption of refined carbohydrates, added sugars, and processed foods, as they can contribute to weight gain and negatively impact overall health.

Choosing nutrient-dense carbohydrates, incorporating them into balanced meals, and pairing them with proteins and healthy fats can support healthy weight management and overall well-being.

In conclusion, carbohydrates are an essential source of energy and play a vital role in overall health and vitality. Understanding the different types of carbohydrates, their effects on blood sugar levels, and their contributions to nutrient intake can help individuals make informed choices and support their health and wellness goals. By incorporating smart carbohydrates into a balanced and varied diet, individuals can fuel their bodies, maintain stable energy levels, and support overall health and vitality.

Chapter 4: Essential Fats for a Healthy Body and Mind

4.1 The Importance of Dietary Fats

Dietary fats are an essential macronutrient that provides energy, supports cell structure, and aids in the absorption of fat-soluble vitamins (A, D, E, and K). Fats are composed of fatty acids, which are long chains of carbon atoms. The body can synthesize some fatty acids, but others, known as essential fatty acids, must be obtained from the diet.

Fats are a concentrated source of energy, providing nine calories per gram, compared to four calories per gram from carbohydrates and proteins. They serve as a stored energy reserve, helping the body maintain energy levels during times of fasting or low food intake.

It is essential to include a variety of dietary fats in the diet to support overall health and well-being. However, not all fats are created equal, and the types and amounts of fats consumed can impact health outcomes.

4.2 Types of Fats: Saturated, Unsaturated, and Trans Fats

Fats can be classified into three main types based on their chemical structure: saturated, unsaturated, and trans fats.

Saturated fats are fats in which all carbon atoms are bonded to hydrogen atoms and have no double bonds between carbon atoms. They are typically solid at room temperature and are found in animal products like meat, dairy, and butter, as well as in tropical oils like coconut and palm oil. High intake of saturated fats has been linked to increased LDL cholesterol levels and a higher risk of heart disease.

Unsaturated fats, on the other hand, have one or more double bonds between carbon atoms, which causes them to be liquid at room temperature. They are divided into monounsaturated and polyunsaturated fats. Monounsaturated fats are found in olive oil, avocados, and nuts, while polyunsaturated fats include omega-3 and omega-6 fatty acids, found in fatty fish, flaxseeds, and vegetable oils. Unsaturated fats have been associated with improved heart health and reduced risk of chronic diseases when consumed in place of saturated and trans fats.

Trans fats are a type of unsaturated fat that has undergone a process called hydrogenation to improve shelf life and stability. Trans fats are often found in partially hydrogenated oils used in processed and fried foods, baked goods, and margarine. Consumption of trans fats has been strongly linked to an increased risk of heart disease and other adverse health effects.

4.3 Omega-3 and Omega-6 Fatty Acids

Omega-3 and omega-6 fatty acids are polyunsaturated fats that play crucial roles in the body's inflammatory response, blood clotting, and cell membrane structure. While both types are essential for health, the balance between omega-3 and omega-6 intake is essential.

Omega-3 fatty acids, found primarily in fatty fish (such as salmon, mackerel, and sardines), flaxseeds, chia seeds, and walnuts, are anti-inflammatory and are associated with heart health benefits. They are especially important for brain function, cognitive health, and reducing the risk of cardiovascular disease.

Omega-6 fatty acids are found in vegetable oils (such as corn, soybean, and sunflower oil) and many processed foods. While they are also essential, excessive omega-6 intake relative to omega-3 can promote inflammation and increase the risk of chronic diseases.

Balancing the intake of omega-3 and omega-6 fatty acids is essential for optimal health. A diet rich in fatty fish, nuts, and seeds can provide adequate omega-3 while limiting processed foods high in omega-6 fatty acids.

4.4 Sources of Healthy Fats: Nuts, Seeds, and Avocado

Nuts, seeds, and avocado are excellent sources of healthy fats, providing a range of nutrients and health benefits.

Nuts, such as almonds, walnuts, and pistachios, are rich in monounsaturated fats, which have been associated with heart health benefits. They also contain fiber, vitamins, minerals, and antioxidants. Consuming nuts regularly has been linked to a reduced risk of heart disease and improved cholesterol levels.

Seeds, including flaxseeds, chia seeds, and hemp seeds, are particularly high in omega-3 fatty acids. These seeds also provide fiber, protein, and micronutrients like magnesium and calcium. They can be easily incorporated into the diet by adding them to smoothies, yogurt, salads, or oatmeal.

Avocado is a unique fruit that is rich in monounsaturated fats and provides a creamy texture to dishes. Avocado consumption has been associated with improved heart health, reduced inflammation, and better absorption of fat-soluble vitamins.

Incorporating nuts, seeds, and avocado into the diet is a tasty and nutritious way to increase healthy fat intake and support overall health.

4.5 Benefits of Fish Oil for Heart Health and Inflammation

Fish oil is a popular supplement that is rich in omega-3 fatty acids, particularly eicosapentaenoic acid (EPA) and docosahexaenoic acid

(DHA). Consuming fish oil or incorporating fatty fish into the diet has been linked to numerous health benefits.

Fish oil is well-known for its positive impact on heart health. It has been shown to reduce triglyceride levels, lower blood pressure, and improve blood vessel function. These effects contribute to a reduced risk of heart disease and stroke.

Omega-3 fatty acids in fish oil also possess potent anti-inflammatory properties. Chronic inflammation is a key driver of many diseases, including cardiovascular disease, autoimmune conditions, and certain types of cancer. By reducing inflammation

, fish oil may help prevent or alleviate these conditions.

Fish oil may also benefit cognitive function and mental health. DHA, one of the omega-3 fatty acids in fish oil, is a crucial component of brain cell membranes and plays a role in brain development and function. Adequate DHA intake has been associated with a lower risk of cognitive decline and improved mood.

While fish oil supplements can be beneficial, it is essential to obtain omega-3 fatty acids from a variety of sources, including fatty fish and plant-based options like flaxseeds and chia seeds.

4.6 Cooking Oils and Their Impact on Health

Cooking oils play a significant role in food preparation, but not all oils are equally healthy. The choice of cooking oil can impact nutrient intake, flavor, and the formation of harmful compounds when exposed to high heat.

Some cooking oils, like olive oil and avocado oil, are rich in monounsaturated fats and have a high smoke point, making them suitable for high-heat cooking methods like sautéing and roasting.

Other oils, such as coconut oil and butter, have a lower smoke point and are better suited for medium-heat cooking. While coconut oil is a source of saturated fat, some studies suggest that it may have a neutral effect on heart health when used in moderation.

It is essential to avoid using oils with low smoke points, such as flaxseed oil and walnut oil, for cooking at high temperatures, as they can become rancid and lose their nutritional value.

Incorporating a variety of cooking oils into the diet can provide a balance of healthy fats and contribute to flavorful and nutritious meals.

4.7 Fats for Brain Health and Cognitive Function

Fat plays a vital role in brain health and cognitive function. The brain is composed of nearly 60% fat, and specific fats, such as omega-3 fatty acids, are particularly important for brain development and function.

DHA, an omega-3 fatty acid abundant in fish oil, is a crucial component of cell membranes in the brain. It supports communication between brain cells and is essential for learning, memory, and cognitive performance.

Consuming omega-3 fatty acids from fish oil or plant-based sources like flaxseeds and walnuts has been associated with a lower risk of cognitive decline and age-related cognitive impairment.

In addition to omega-3 fatty acids, other fats, such as monounsaturated fats found in olive oil and avocados, have been linked to better cognitive function and a reduced risk of neurodegenerative diseases like Alzheimer's.

A diet rich in a variety of healthy fats can support brain health and cognitive function throughout life.

4.8 Fat and Hormonal Balance

Fats play a crucial role in hormonal balance, as certain hormones, like estrogen and testosterone, are synthesized from cholesterol, a type of fat.

Adequate fat intake is necessary for hormone production, especially for women's reproductive hormones. Low-fat diets or diets that restrict healthy fats may negatively impact hormonal balance and menstrual cycles.

Omega-3 fatty acids, in particular, have been associated with reduced menstrual pain and may help alleviate symptoms of premenstrual syndrome (PMS) in some women.

Balancing fat intake, including omega-3 and omega-6 fatty acids, can support hormonal health and overall well-being.

4.9 Dietary Fat and Weight Management

Contrary to the misconception that fat intake leads to weight gain, dietary fats can play a beneficial role in weight management when chosen wisely.

Fats are more calorie-dense than carbohydrates and proteins, which can make it easy to overconsume them. However, fats can also promote satiety, helping individuals feel fuller for longer and potentially reducing overall calorie intake.

Healthy fats, such as monounsaturated and polyunsaturated fats found in nuts, seeds, and fatty fish, can be included in a balanced diet to support weight loss and weight maintenance. These fats can provide sustained energy and prevent overeating, which may occur with low-fat diets.

On the other hand, it is essential to limit the intake of unhealthy fats, such as trans fats and excessive saturated fats, as they can contribute to weight gain and adverse health effects.

Balancing fat intake and considering portion sizes can support weight management goals and overall health.

4.10 Practical Tips for Incorporating Healthy Fats into Your Diet

Incorporating healthy fats into the diet can be enjoyable and straightforward with some practical tips:

- Add a serving of nuts or seeds to your morning oatmeal or yogurt for a nutrient-rich breakfast.

- Use olive oil or avocado oil in salad dressings and marinades to add flavor and healthy fats to your meals.

- Snack on a handful of almonds or walnuts for a satisfying and nourishing snack.

- Enjoy fatty fish like salmon or mackerel at least twice a week for a boost of omega-3 fatty acids.

- Include avocado slices in sandwiches, wraps, or salads for a creamy and nutritious addition.

- Make your own trail mix with a mix of nuts, seeds, and dried fruits for a convenient on-the-go snack.

   - Use nut butters like almond butter or peanut butter as a dip for apple slices or celery sticks.

By incorporating a variety of healthy fats into your daily meals and snacks, you can support overall health, enhance flavor in your dishes, and enjoy the many benefits that essential fats offer for your body   and   mind.

Chapter 5: Understanding Vitamins and Minerals

5.1 Water-Soluble Vitamins: B-complex and Vitamin C

Water-soluble vitamins are a group of vitamins that dissolve in water and are not stored in significant amounts in the body. They need to be consumed regularly as any excess is excreted through urine. The two main groups of water-soluble vitamins are the B-complex vitamins and vitamin C.

The B-complex vitamins include B1 (thiamine), B2 (riboflavin), B3 (niacin), B5 (pantothenic acid), B6 (pyridoxine), B7 (biotin), B9 (folate), and B12 (cobalamin). These vitamins play essential roles in energy metabolism, supporting the function of enzymes that are involved in breaking down carbohydrates, proteins, and fats for energy production.

Vitamin C, also known as ascorbic acid, is a powerful antioxidant that helps protect cells from damage caused by free radicals. It is also necessary for collagen synthesis, which is essential for maintaining healthy skin, connective tissues, and wound healing.

Water-soluble vitamins are found in a wide variety of foods, including whole grains, fruits, vegetables, legumes, nuts, and seeds. To ensure an adequate intake of these vitamins, it is essential to consume a diverse and balanced diet.

5.2 Fat-Soluble Vitamins: A, D, E, and K

Fat-soluble vitamins are vitamins that dissolve in fat and are stored in the body's fatty tissues and liver. Unlike water-soluble vitamins, they can be stored for more extended periods, and excess intake can lead to toxicity. The four main fat-soluble vitamins are vitamins A, D, E, and K.

Vitamin A is essential for vision, immune function, and the health of the skin and mucous membranes. It is found in two forms: retinol (preformed vitamin A) from animal sources and beta-carotene (provitamin A) from plant sources. Foods rich in vitamin A include liver, fish oil, sweet potatoes, carrots, spinach, and other leafy greens.

Vitamin D is known as the "sunshine vitamin" because the body can produce it when the skin is exposed to sunlight. It plays a crucial role in calcium absorption and bone health. It is also involved in immune function and may have protective effects against certain diseases. Dietary sources of vitamin D include fatty fish, fortified dairy products, and some mushrooms.

Vitamin E is a powerful antioxidant that helps protect cells from oxidative damage. It is essential for maintaining healthy skin and eyes and supporting the immune system. Nuts, seeds, vegetable oils, and leafy greens are good sources of vitamin E.

Vitamin K is necessary for blood clotting and bone health. There are two primary forms of vitamin K: K1 (phylloquinone), found in leafy green vegetables, and K2 (menaquinone), found in fermented foods and animal products. Adequate vitamin K intake is crucial for proper blood clotting and preventing bone fractures.

As fat-soluble vitamins are stored in the body, it is essential to be mindful of excessive supplementation, as it can lead to toxicity. Consuming a varied diet with a range of nutrient-rich foods can help maintain optimal levels of these vitamins.

5.3 Micronutrients for Bone Health: Calcium, Magnesium, and Vitamin D

Bone health is crucial for overall well-being, and several micronutrients play key roles in supporting healthy bones.

Calcium is the most abundant mineral in the body and is primarily stored in bones and teeth. It is essential for maintaining bone density and strength. Adequate calcium intake throughout life, as part of a well-balanced diet, may help reduce the risk of osteoporosis.

Good sources of calcium include dairy products, leafy greens, almonds, tofu, and fortified plant-based milk.

Magnesium is another essential mineral for bone health. It works in conjunction with calcium and vitamin D to support bone density and structure. Magnesium is involved in over 300 biochemical reactions in the body and plays a role in muscle function, nerve function, and energy production.

Foods rich in magnesium include whole grains, nuts, seeds, legumes, leafy greens, and avocados.

Vitamin D, as mentioned earlier, is essential for calcium absorption and utilization in bones. It helps regulate calcium and phosphorus levels in the blood and promotes the formation of strong bones.

In addition to dietary sources, vitamin D can be synthesized by the body when the skin is exposed to sunlight. However, many people may have insufficient vitamin D levels, especially in regions with limited sunlight exposure or during the winter months. For this reason, supplementation may be necessary, especially for individuals at risk of deficiency.

5.4 Antioxidant Vitamins: Vitamin A, C, and E

Antioxidant vitamins are vitamins that help neutralize free radicals, which are highly reactive molecules that can damage cells and contribute to oxidative stress. The body produces free radicals as part of its natural processes, but factors such as pollution, smoking, and exposure to ultraviolet (UV) radiation can increase their production.

Vitamin A, vitamin C, and vitamin E are potent antioxidants that play essential roles in protecting the body from oxidative damage.

Vitamin A, in the form of retinol and beta-carotene, is crucial for maintaining healthy skin and vision and supporting the immune system.

Vitamin C is an important water-soluble antioxidant that helps protect cells from oxidative stress and supports immune function. It also plays a key role in collagen synthesis, wound healing, and iron absorption.

Vitamin E is a fat-soluble antioxidant that protects cell membranes from damage caused by free radicals. It works synergistically with vitamin C to enhance antioxidant protection.

Including a variety of fruits and vegetables in the diet can provide an abundance of these antioxidant vitamins. Berries, citrus fruits, bell peppers, tomatoes, spinach, and nuts are excellent sources of antioxidants.

5.5 The Role of Vitamin K in Blood Clotting and Bone Health

Vitamin K is a fat-soluble vitamin that is essential for blood clotting and bone health. It is necessary for the activation of specific proteins involved in the coagulation cascade, which helps prevent excessive bleeding when an injury occurs.

There are two primary forms of vitamin K: vitamin K1 (phylloquinone) and vitamin K2 (menaquinone). Vitamin K1 is found in leafy green vegetables, while vitamin K2 is found in fermented foods, certain animal products, and produced by gut bacteria.

In addition to its role in blood clotting, vitamin K is essential for bone health. It helps regulate calcium metabolism and ensures that calcium is deposited in bones and teeth rather than in soft tissues, where it can cause harm.

Adequate vitamin K intake is crucial for maintaining bone density and reducing the risk of fractures. Including leafy greens, broccoli, Brussels sprouts, and fermented foods in the diet can provide an adequate amount of vitamin K.

5.6 Essential Minerals: Iron, Zinc, and Selenium

Iron, zinc, and selenium are essential minerals that play crucial roles in various physiological processes.

Iron is necessary for the production of hemoglobin, a protein in red blood cells that carries oxygen throughout the body. Iron deficiency can lead to anemia, characterized by fatigue, weakness, and decreased immune function.

Good sources of iron include red meat, poultry, fish,

beans, lentils, tofu, and fortified cereals. Vitamin C can enhance iron absorption, so consuming iron-rich foods with vitamin C-rich foods can improve iron uptake.

Zinc is involved in over 300 enzymatic reactions in the body and is crucial for immune function, wound healing, and DNA synthesis. It is also essential for normal growth and development during childhood, adolescence, and pregnancy.

Zinc is found in various foods, including meat, shellfish, legumes, nuts, seeds, and whole grains.

Selenium is a trace mineral that acts as an antioxidant and is involved in thyroid hormone metabolism. Adequate selenium intake is crucial for maintaining a healthy immune system and supporting thyroid function.

Selenium is found in foods such as Brazil nuts, seafood, meat, and whole grains.

5.7 Iodine for Thyroid Function

Iodine is an essential trace mineral that plays a critical role in thyroid function. The thyroid gland uses iodine to produce thyroid hormones, which are essential for regulating metabolism, energy production, and overall growth and development.

Iodine deficiency can lead to a condition called goiter, which is characterized by an enlarged thyroid gland. Severe iodine deficiency during pregnancy can lead to cognitive and developmental issues in the offspring, a condition known as cretinism.

Iodine is naturally found in iodized salt, seafood, seaweed, and dairy products. In regions where iodine deficiency is common, iodized salt is an effective strategy to prevent deficiency.

5.8 Chromium and Blood Sugar Regulation

Chromium is a trace mineral that plays a role in blood sugar regulation. It enhances the action of insulin, a hormone that helps transport glucose into cells, where it can be used for energy.

Chromium is found in small amounts in a variety of foods, including whole grains, meat, poultry, fish, and some fruits and vegetables.

While chromium deficiency is rare, adequate intake is essential for maintaining stable blood sugar levels and supporting overall metabolic health.

5.9 The Power of Phytonutrients and Plant Compounds

Phytonutrients are naturally occurring compounds found in plants that have beneficial effects on human health. They are not considered essential nutrients like vitamins and minerals, but research has shown that they play vital roles in disease prevention and overall well-being.

Phytonutrients act as antioxidants, anti-inflammatory agents, and support various body functions. Some well-known phytonutrients include flavonoids, carotenoids, polyphenols, and plant sterols.

Flavonoids are found in fruits, vegetables, and herbs, and they have been linked to reduced risk of heart disease and certain cancers.

Carotenoids, like beta-carotene found in carrots and lycopene in tomatoes, are antioxidants that help protect cells from oxidative damage.

Polyphenols, present in foods like berries, tea, and cocoa, have anti-inflammatory and antioxidant properties that can support cardiovascular health.

Plant sterols, found in nuts, seeds, and vegetable oils, can help lower LDL cholesterol levels and support heart health.

Incorporating a wide variety of colorful fruits and vegetables, as well as herbs, spices, nuts, and seeds, can provide a diverse array of phytonutrients and enhance overall health.

5.10 Balancing Vitamin and Mineral Intake Through Diet

Achieving a balanced intake of vitamins and minerals is best achieved through a varied and nutritious diet. A diet rich in fruits, vegetables, whole grains, nuts, seeds, lean proteins, and healthy fats can provide a wide range of essential nutrients.

Balancing vitamin and mineral intake involves paying attention to nutrient-dense foods and avoiding excessive reliance on processed and refined foods that may lack essential nutrients.

Individual nutrient needs may vary based on age, sex, life stage, and health status. Consulting with a registered dietitian or healthcare professional can help determine specific nutrient needs and create a personalized dietary plan to ensure optimal vitamin and mineral intake.

By understanding the roles of vitamins and minerals and making informed food choices, individuals can support their overall health and   well-being.

Chapter 6: Hydration and Its Impact on Health

6.1 The Importance of Staying Hydrated

Staying hydrated is essential for overall health and well-being. Water is a fundamental component of the human body, making up about 60% of an adult's body weight. It plays a crucial role in various physiological processes, including temperature regulation, nutrient transport, waste removal, and lubrication of joints.

Maintaining proper hydration is vital for supporting optimal organ function, cognitive performance, and physical endurance. Adequate hydration helps regulate blood pressure, heart rate, and electrolyte balance.

Hydration needs can vary based on factors such as age, sex, activity level, and environmental conditions. Ensuring sufficient fluid intake is essential to prevent dehydration, which can lead to a range of health issues, including fatigue, impaired cognitive function, and even heat-related illnesses in extreme cases.

6.2 Water and Its Role in the Body

Water is the primary component of cells, tissues, and organs throughout the body. It is involved in numerous physiological processes, including:

- Transporting nutrients and oxygen to cells and removing waste products from the body.
- Regulating body temperature through sweating and evaporation.
- Lubricating joints, reducing friction between bones.
- Supporting digestion by aiding in the breakdown of food and the absorption of nutrients.
- Cushioning and protecting vital organs, such as the brain and spinal cord.

Water is essential for maintaining overall health, and its consumption is the most effective way to stay hydrated. Other beverages and foods can contribute to hydration, but pure water remains the best choice for ensuring proper fluid balance in the body.

6.3 Signs and Symptoms of Dehydration

Dehydration occurs when the body loses more fluids than it takes in, leading to an insufficient amount of water to carry out essential functions. Mild dehydration can cause symptoms such as thirst, dry mouth, and dark yellow urine. Other signs of dehydration include fatigue, dizziness, headache, and reduced urine output.

As dehydration worsens, it can lead to more severe symptoms, including confusion, rapid heartbeat, sunken eyes, and low blood pressure. Severe dehydration is a medical emergency and requires immediate attention.

Infants, young children, older adults, and individuals with certain medical conditions are particularly vulnerable to dehydration and may need extra attention to their fluid intake.

6.4 Electrolytes: Sodium, Potassium, and Magnesium

Electrolytes are minerals that carry an electric charge in the body. The main electrolytes involved in hydration are sodium, potassium, and magnesium.

Sodium and potassium are essential for maintaining the body's fluid balance. Sodium helps retain water in the body, while potassium works in conjunction with sodium to regulate fluid levels inside and outside cells. Adequate sodium and potassium intake is crucial for proper muscle function, nerve transmission, and heart health.

Magnesium also plays a role in maintaining proper hydration by influencing the movement of water and electrolytes in and out of cells. It is involved in many enzymatic reactions in the body and supports muscle function, nerve function, and bone health.

Electrolyte imbalances can occur with dehydration or excessive fluid loss through sweating. Replenishing electrolytes through balanced meals and, in some cases, electrolyte-rich beverages or supplements can help maintain optimal hydration and prevent electrolyte disturbances.

6.5 Hydration for Athletes and Active Individuals

Hydration is particularly important for athletes and individuals engaged in physical activity. During exercise, the body loses water through sweat to help regulate body temperature. Proper hydration before, during, and after exercise is essential for performance, endurance, and recovery.

Hydration needs for athletes can vary depending on factors such as the intensity and duration of exercise, sweat rate, and environmental conditions. Drinking water or electrolyte-rich beverages during exercise can help replace fluids and maintain electrolyte balance.

Additionally, consuming carbohydrates and electrolytes during prolonged or intense exercise can provide a source of energy and support optimal performance.

Athletes should monitor their fluid intake and consider individual factors to develop a personalized hydration plan that meets their specific needs.

6.6 Hydration During Pregnancy and Lactation

Pregnant and breastfeeding women have increased fluid needs to support their own physiological changes and the needs of their growing baby or nursing child.

During pregnancy, proper hydration is essential for adequate blood volume, nutrient transport to the placenta, and proper amniotic fluid levels. Pregnant women should aim to drink plenty of water and other hydrating beverages throughout the day.

Similarly, breastfeeding women should prioritize hydration to support milk production and ensure the milk is rich in nutrients.

For pregnant and breastfeeding women, listening to their body's thirst cues and maintaining a balanced diet with a variety of hydrating foods and beverages is crucial for meeting increased fluid needs.

6.7 Hydration and Cognitive Function

Proper hydration has a significant impact on cognitive function. Even mild dehydration can impair concentration, memory, and mental alertness.

Studies have shown that dehydration can lead to reduced cognitive performance, including decreased attention, slower reaction times, and impaired short-term memory.

Maintaining adequate hydration throughout the day is essential for supporting optimal brain function, focus, and productivity.

6.8 The Role of Fluids in Digestion

Hydration plays a crucial role in the digestive process. Water helps break down food, dissolve nutrients, and facilitate the absorption of nutrients in the intestines.

Adequate fluid intake supports regular bowel movements and prevents constipation. Insufficient hydration can lead to harder stools and difficulty passing waste, contributing to constipation and discomfort.

Drinking enough water and staying hydrated can help maintain digestive health and support the efficient breakdown and absorption of nutrients.

6.9 Different Sources of Hydration: Water, Herbal Teas, and Infusions

While water is the most effective way to stay hydrated, other beverages can contribute to fluid intake as well.

Herbal teas are a hydrating option that provides additional health benefits from the herbs and spices used. Herbal teas are caffeine-free and can be enjoyed hot or cold.

Infused water, made by adding fruits, vegetables, or herbs to water, can enhance the taste and appeal of plain water, making it more enjoyable to drink.

Fruits and vegetables with high water content, such as watermelon, cucumber, and oranges, can also contribute to hydration and provide additional vitamins and minerals.

It is essential to be mindful of added sugars and excessive caffeine intake in certain beverages, as they can impact hydration levels. Opting for hydrating beverages without added sugars or caffeine is the best choice for overall health.

6.10 Tips for Maintaining Optimal Hydration

To maintain optimal hydration throughout the day, consider the following tips:

1. Carry a reusable water bottle and sip water throughout the day, even if you don't feel thirsty.

2. Pay attention to your body's thirst cues and drink water when you feel thirsty.

3. Monitor your urine color - a pale yellow color indicates adequate hydration, while darker urine may indicate the need for more fluids.

4. Incorporate hydrating foods, such as fruits and vegetables with high water content, into your diet.

5. Set reminders to drink water, especially during busy or active periods when it's easy to forget.

6. For athletes or those engaged in physical activity, drink fluids before, during, and after exercise to stay hydrated.

7. Avoid excessive consumption of caffeinated and alcoholic beverages, as they can contribute to dehydration.

8. Consider flavoring water with fresh fruit, herbs, or cucumber slices for added taste appeal.

9. Be mindful of environmental factors that can increase fluid needs, such as hot weather

or high altitudes.

10. Listen to your body and adjust your fluid intake based on individual needs and circumstances.

By prioritizing hydration and making conscious efforts to maintain fluid balance, individuals can support their overall health, well-being, and optimal body functioning. Remember, water is a precious resource for our bodies, and staying adequately hydrated is a simple yet powerful way to promote good health.

Chapter 7: Sodium and Potassium - Finding the Balance

7.1 Sodium: Understanding the Sodium-Potassium Pump

Sodium and potassium are essential electrolytes that play crucial roles in maintaining various physiological functions in the body. One of the most vital processes involving these minerals is the sodium-potassium pump, a mechanism that helps maintain the cell's resting membrane potential and facilitates nerve impulses and muscle contractions.

The sodium-potassium pump is an active transport system found in cell membranes throughout the body. It regulates the balance of sodium and potassium ions inside and outside the cells, creating an electrical gradient necessary for cellular communication.

During the pumping process, the pump actively transports three sodium ions out of the cell while bringing two potassium ions into the cell. This creates an electrochemical gradient, contributing to the cell's resting membrane potential. This potential is essential for proper nerve function, muscle contractions, and overall cell communication.

Maintaining the sodium-potassium pump's balance is crucial for optimal cellular function, nerve transmission, and muscle contraction. Adequate intake of both sodium and potassium is necessary to support this delicate balance and ensure overall health.

7.2 Sodium's Impact on Blood Pressure

Sodium is an essential mineral that plays a role in regulating blood pressure and fluid balance in the body. When sodium is consumed in excess, it can lead to an increase in extracellular fluid volume, resulting in elevated blood pressure.

High blood pressure, also known as hypertension, is a significant risk factor for cardiovascular diseases, including heart attack, stroke, and kidney disease. Reducing sodium intake is one of the key dietary interventions to manage and prevent hypertension.

The link between sodium intake and blood pressure is particularly sensitive in certain individuals, such as those with a genetic predisposition to salt sensitivity. For such individuals, even a moderate increase in sodium intake can have a substantial impact on blood pressure.

To manage blood pressure effectively, it is essential to consume a balanced diet with a focus on whole, minimally processed foods and limit the intake of sodium-rich processed and packaged foods.

7.3 The Dangers of Excessive Sodium Intake

While sodium is necessary for various bodily functions, excessive sodium intake can have adverse effects on health.

One of the primary concerns associated with high sodium intake is hypertension, as discussed earlier. Prolonged high blood pressure can strain the heart and blood vessels, increasing the risk of cardiovascular diseases.

Excessive sodium intake can also lead to fluid retention, causing bloating and swelling, particularly in the hands, feet, and ankles. This can be particularly problematic for individuals with heart or kidney conditions.

Additionally, high sodium intake may contribute to kidney stones and reduce calcium excretion, potentially leading to a negative impact on bone health.

Furthermore, high sodium intake has been associated with an increased risk of stomach cancer, as it can irritate the stomach lining and promote inflammation.

Reducing sodium intake through dietary modifications and reading food labels to identify hidden sources of sodium in processed foods can help mitigate these health risks.

7.4 Reducing Sodium in Your Diet

Reducing sodium intake can be achieved through several dietary strategies:

1. Choose whole, unprocessed foods: Fresh fruits, vegetables, lean proteins, and whole grains naturally contain lower amounts of sodium compared to processed foods.

2. Limit processed and packaged foods: Many processed foods, such as canned soups, sauces, snacks, and condiments, are high in sodium. Opt for low-sodium or no-salt-added versions, or better yet, make homemade alternatives.

3. Use herbs and spices: Instead of relying on salt for flavor, experiment with herbs, spices, and citrus to add taste to your meals.

4. Rinse canned foods: If using canned beans or vegetables, rinse them thoroughly under water to reduce their sodium content.

5. Cook at home: Preparing meals at home allows you to control the amount of sodium added to your dishes.

6. Read food labels: Be mindful of sodium content listed on food labels and aim to choose products with lower sodium levels.

7.5 Potassium's Role in Heart Health

Potassium is a crucial mineral that plays a significant role in heart health. It is essential for maintaining the heart's electrical activity, ensuring proper heartbeat and rhythm.

Potassium helps balance sodium levels in the body, promoting healthy blood pressure. Adequate potassium intake can counteract the negative effects of high sodium consumption on blood pressure.

Furthermore, potassium supports the relaxation of blood vessels, improving blood flow and cardiovascular function.

Consuming an adequate amount of potassium-rich foods can be beneficial for heart health, reducing the risk of cardiovascular diseases and stroke.

7.6 Potassium-Rich Foods: Bananas, Sweet Potatoes, and Spinach

A diet rich in potassium can be achieved by incorporating a variety of potassium-rich foods into daily meals:

Bananas: Bananas are a well-known source of potassium, providing around 400-450 mg per medium-sized banana.

Sweet Potatoes: Sweet potatoes are not only delicious but also a great source of potassium, with approximately 450-500 mg per medium-sized sweet potato.

Spinach: Dark leafy greens like spinach are rich in potassium, offering around 500-600 mg per cooked cup.

Oranges: Citrus fruits, including oranges, are excellent sources of potassium, providing approximately 230-250 mg per medium-sized orange.

Avocados: Avocados are not only rich in healthy fats but also a good source of potassium, with around 700-900 mg per medium-sized avocado.

Tomatoes: Tomatoes are versatile and provide about 250-300 mg of potassium per medium-sized tomato.

Beans and Lentils: Legumes, such as beans and lentils, are rich in potassium, offering approximately 400-600 mg per cooked cup.

Potassium-rich foods can be easily incorporated into various dishes, including salads, smoothies, soups, and main courses.

7.7 Balancing Sodium and Potassium for Electrolyte Health

Maintaining a balance between sodium and potassium intake is crucial for overall electrolyte health. Both minerals play complementary roles in fluid balance, nerve function, and muscle contractions.

A high sodium-to-potassium ratio, as often seen in diets rich in processed foods and low in fruits and vegetables, can disrupt the sodium-potassium pump's balance and contribute to high blood pressure and cardiovascular issues.

Balancing sodium and potassium intake can be achieved by:

1. Reducing sodium intake from processed and packaged foods.

2. Increasing potassium-rich foods in the diet, as mentioned in the previous section.

3. Choosing a diet rich in whole, minimally processed foods.

A diet focused on whole, nutrient-dense foods can naturally support an appropriate balance of sodium and potassium intake.

7.8 Sodium and Potassium Requirements for Athletes

Athletes have unique hydration and electrolyte needs due to increased fluid losses through sweat during physical activity. Proper hydration and electrolyte balance are crucial for maintaining performance and preventing dehydration and muscle cramps.

Both sodium and potassium are lost through sweat during exercise, and these losses must be adequately replenished to support optimal athletic performance.

Athletes should focus on consuming a balanced diet with sufficient potassium-rich foods and, in some cases, electrolyte-rich beverages during and after exercise to replace lost fluids and minerals.

For individuals engaged in intense or prolonged exercise, sports drinks or electrolyte supplements may be beneficial. However, it is essential to choose options with balanced sodium and potassium levels and to avoid excessive consumption of sugary sports drinks.

7.9 Hidden Sources of Sodium in Processed Foods

Sodium is a prevalent ingredient

in processed foods due to its flavor-enhancing properties and preservative qualities. It can be challenging to identify hidden sources of sodium in the diet, as many processed foods contain high amounts of added salt.

Some common hidden sources of sodium include:

- Processed meats: Deli meats, bacon, sausages, and hot dogs are often high in sodium.
    - Canned soups and broths: Canned soups and broths can be significant sources of sodium, even those labeled as "low-sodium."
    - Condiments: Sauces, dressings, and condiments like soy sauce, ketchup, and salad dressings can be surprisingly high in sodium.
    - Packaged snacks: Chips, crackers, and pretzels often contain added salt.

- Cheese: Some types of cheese, especially processed cheese and certain varieties of feta and blue cheese, can be high in sodium.

Reading food labels and choosing products with lower sodium content or opting for homemade alternatives can help reduce sodium intake from hidden sources.

7.10 Monitoring Sodium and Potassium Intake for Optimal Health

Monitoring sodium and potassium intake is essential for maintaining overall health, particularly heart health and electrolyte balance.

Tracking sodium intake involves being mindful of the sodium content in processed foods and choosing lower-sodium alternatives. It is also essential to balance sodium intake with potassium-rich foods to support overall electrolyte health.

Keeping a food diary or using nutrition apps can help individuals become more aware of their sodium and potassium intake and identify areas for improvement in their dietary habits.

For individuals with specific health conditions, such as hypertension or kidney issues, consulting with a registered dietitian can provide personalized guidance on managing sodium and potassium intake.

By finding the right balance between sodium and potassium intake and making conscious dietary choices, individuals can support their cardiovascular health, maintain proper fluid balance, and ensure optimal electrolyte function for overall well-being.

Chapter 8: Fiber - A Key Component for Digestive Health

8.1 The Importance of Dietary Fiber

Dietary fiber is a type of carbohydrate that the human body cannot digest or absorb. Despite its indigestibility, fiber plays a crucial role in supporting digestive health and overall well-being.

Fiber is classified into two main types: soluble fiber and insoluble fiber. Both types of fiber offer unique health benefits and contribute to various aspects of digestive health.

Unlike other carbohydrates, fiber passes through the digestive system relatively intact, adding bulk to stools and facilitating regular bowel movements. Adequate fiber intake is associated with a reduced risk of constipation and other gastrointestinal issues.

Beyond its effects on digestion, fiber also influences blood sugar regulation, heart health, weight management, and gut microbiota composition. Including a variety of fiber-rich foods in the diet is essential for promoting overall health and preventing certain chronic diseases.

8.2 Soluble vs. Insoluble Fiber

Soluble fiber and insoluble fiber are the two main types of dietary fiber, each with distinct properties and health benefits.

Soluble Fiber:
- Soluble fiber dissolves in water and forms a gel-like substance in the digestive tract.
- This type of fiber helps slow down the absorption of nutrients, including sugars and cholesterol, leading to better blood sugar and cholesterol management.
- Foods rich in soluble fiber include oats, barley, legumes (beans and lentils), apples, citrus fruits, and flaxseeds.

Insoluble Fiber:
- Insoluble fiber does not dissolve in water and retains its form throughout the digestive process.
- This type of fiber adds bulk to stools, helping to prevent and alleviate constipation.
- Foods rich in insoluble fiber include whole grains (wheat bran, whole wheat, brown rice), nuts, seeds, and many vegetables like broccoli and carrots.

Both types of fiber are essential for a well-balanced diet and optimal digestive health. It is best to consume a variety of fiber-rich foods to benefit from the unique properties of each type of fiber.

8.3 Benefits of Fiber for Digestion

Fiber offers a range of benefits for digestion and gastrointestinal health:

- Constipation Prevention: Insoluble fiber adds bulk to stools, promoting regular bowel movements and reducing the risk of constipation.
- Diverticular Disease Prevention: Adequate fiber intake is associated with a lower risk of diverticular disease, a condition characterized by pouches forming in the colon wall.
- Hemorrhoid Prevention: A high-fiber diet can help prevent and alleviate hemorrhoids, which are swollen blood vessels in the rectal area.
- Colon Cancer Prevention: Some studies suggest that a diet rich in fiber may lower the risk of colon cancer, although more research is needed to establish a definitive link.
- Improved Gut Health: Fiber serves as a prebiotic, promoting the growth of beneficial gut bacteria and supporting a healthy gut microbiome.
- Detoxification: Soluble fiber can bind to certain toxins and remove them from the body, supporting natural detoxification processes.

8.4 High-Fiber Foods: Whole Grains, Legumes, and Fruits

To ensure an adequate intake of fiber, incorporating high-fiber foods into the diet is essential. Some excellent sources of fiber include:

Whole Grains:

- Whole grains like oats, barley, quinoa, brown rice, and whole wheat are rich in fiber, vitamins, and minerals.

- Choose whole grain options for bread, pasta, and cereals to increase fiber intake.

Legumes:

- Beans, lentils, chickpeas, and peas are high in both soluble and insoluble fiber.

- Including legumes in soups, salads, and stews is an excellent way to boost fiber content.

Fruits:

- Many fruits are excellent sources of fiber, especially when consumed with their skin.

- Apples, pears, berries, oranges, and bananas are among the fruits with higher fiber content.

Vegetables:

- Vegetables like broccoli, Brussels sprouts, carrots, and sweet potatoes are rich in fiber.

- Aim to include a variety of colorful vegetables in your meals to maximize fiber intake.

Nuts and Seeds:

- Almonds, chia seeds, flaxseeds, and sunflower seeds are fiber-rich additions to meals and snacks.

By incorporating these high-fiber foods into daily meals, individuals can increase their fiber intake and support digestive health.

8.5 Fiber and Gut Microbiota

The gut microbiota, also known as gut flora, refers to the trillions of microorganisms living in the gastrointestinal tract. These microorganisms play a crucial role in digestion, nutrient absorption, immune function, and even mood regulation.

Fiber-rich foods serve as prebiotics, providing nourishment for beneficial gut bacteria. When gut bacteria ferment dietary fiber, they produce short-chain fatty acids (SCFAs), such as acetate, propionate, and butyrate.

SCFAs have several health benefits, including reducing inflammation, supporting the gut lining, and influencing the immune system. They also contribute to the production of energy for colon cells and help maintain a healthy gut environment.

Including a variety of fiber-rich foods in the diet is essential for promoting a diverse and balanced gut microbiota, contributing to improved gut health and overall well-being.

8.6 Fiber's Role in Weight Management

Fiber-rich foods play a significant role in weight management due to their effects on satiety, blood sugar regulation, and calorie absorption.

Satiety: Foods high in fiber tend to be more filling, promoting a feeling of fullness and reducing overall calorie intake. This can aid in weight management by reducing the likelihood of overeating.

Blood Sugar Regulation: Soluble fiber slows down the absorption of sugars, leading to more stable blood sugar levels. This can help prevent sharp spikes and crashes in blood sugar, reducing cravings for sugary foods and supporting weight management.

Calorie Absorption: Some of the calories in fiber-rich foods may not be fully absorbed during digestion. Instead, they pass through the digestive tract and are excreted. This can lead to a lower net calorie intake from fiber-containing foods.

Incorporating fiber-rich foods into meals can support weight management efforts by promoting feelings of fullness and reducing overall calorie intake.

8.7 Fiber and Heart Health

Fiber-rich foods are associated with several heart health benefits:

Cholesterol Management: Soluble fiber can help lower LDL cholesterol levels (the "bad" cholesterol) by binding to cholesterol in the digestive tract and promoting its excretion.

Blood Pressure Regulation: Some research suggests that a high-fiber diet may help reduce blood pressure, contributing to heart health.

Reduced Heart Disease Risk: Diets rich in fiber have been linked to a lower risk of heart disease and cardiovascular events.

Inflammation Reduction: The anti-inflammatory properties of fiber may support heart health by reducing chronic inflammation.

By including fiber-rich foods in the diet, individuals can support heart health and reduce the risk of heart disease.

8.8 Getting Enough Fiber on a Plant-Based Diet

Plant-based diets are naturally high in fiber, as they rely primarily on fruits, vegetables, whole grains, legumes, nuts, and seeds. However, some individuals on plant-based diets may need to pay attention to their fiber intake to ensure they are meeting their daily needs.

To get enough fiber on a plant-based diet:

Diversify Plant Foods: Consume a wide variety of fruits, vegetables, whole grains, legumes, nuts, and seeds to maximize fiber intake.

Opt for Whole Foods: Choose whole, minimally processed plant foods to retain their natural

fiber content.

Gradual Increase: If transitioning to a plant-based diet, gradually increase fiber intake to allow the gut to adapt.

Stay Hydrated: Ensure adequate hydration to support healthy digestion and prevent constipation.

Monitor Symptoms: Pay attention to how your body responds to increased fiber intake and adjust as needed.

By being mindful of fiber-rich plant foods and maintaining a balanced diet, individuals on plant-based diets can easily meet their fiber requirements.

8.9 Fiber for Blood Sugar Regulation

Fiber-rich foods can play a significant role in blood sugar regulation, especially for individuals with diabetes or those at risk of developing diabetes.

Soluble fiber slows down the absorption of sugars in the bloodstream, preventing rapid spikes in blood glucose levels after meals. This can help individuals with diabetes manage their blood sugar levels more effectively.

Including fiber-rich foods in meals can also promote a more gradual release of energy, leading to improved energy levels and reduced hunger between meals.

Individuals with diabetes should work with their healthcare provider or a registered dietitian to develop a personalized meal plan that incorporates fiber-rich foods and supports blood sugar management.

8.10 Practical Tips for Increasing Fiber Intake

Increasing fiber intake is relatively simple and can be achieved through various dietary adjustments:

- Gradual Increase: Gradually increase fiber intake to give your digestive system time to adapt.
    - Choose Whole Grains: Opt for whole grain versions of bread, pasta, and cereals to increase fiber content.
    - Include Legumes: Add beans, lentils, and chickpeas to salads, soups, and stews for an easy fiber boost.
    - Snack on Fruits and Vegetables: Incorporate fruits and vegetables into snacks to increase fiber intake between meals.
    - Snack on Nuts and Seeds: Snack on a handful of nuts or seeds for a satisfying and fiber-rich snack.

- Add Fiber to Smoothies: Blend in vegetables like spinach or fruits with their skin into smoothies to boost fiber content.

- Substitute White Rice and Pasta: Replace white rice and pasta with brown rice, quinoa, or whole wheat pasta for higher fiber content.

- Read Labels: Pay attention to food labels and choose products with higher fiber content.

By making these simple dietary changes and including a variety of fiber-rich foods, individuals can easily increase their fiber intake and reap the numerous health benefits of dietary fiber.

Chapter 9: The Power of Antioxidants for Cellular Health

9.1 Understanding Oxidative Stress and Free Radicals

Oxidative stress is a natural process that occurs in the body when there is an imbalance between free radicals and antioxidants. Free radicals are highly reactive molecules that contain unpaired electrons, making them unstable. As a result, they can cause damage to cells, including proteins, lipids, and DNA.

Free radicals are generated as by-products of various physiological processes, such as metabolism, immune response, and detoxification. External factors such as pollution, radiation, cigarette smoke, and certain medications can also contribute to increased free radical production.

In small amounts, free radicals play a role in cell signaling and immune defense. However, excessive levels of free radicals can lead to oxidative stress, which is associated with various health issues, including inflammation, aging, and chronic diseases such as cancer, cardiovascular diseases, and neurodegenerative disorders.

To counteract the harmful effects of free radicals, the body relies on antioxidants. Antioxidants are molecules that neutralize free radicals by donating electrons to stabilize them. They play a critical role in maintaining cellular health and protecting the body from oxidative damage.

9.2 Antioxidants: Vitamins A, C, E, and Selenium

Antioxidants are present in various forms, including vitamins, minerals, and phytonutrients. Some of the most well-known antioxidants include vitamins A, C, E, and the mineral selenium.

Vitamin A: Vitamin A is essential for vision, immune function, and cellular growth. As an antioxidant, it helps protect cells from oxidative damage and supports healthy skin and mucous membranes. Good sources of vitamin A include carrots, sweet potatoes, spinach, and liver.

Vitamin C: Vitamin C is a potent water-soluble antioxidant that plays a crucial role in immune function and collagen synthesis. It helps protect against free radical damage and supports overall cellular health. Citrus fruits, berries, kiwi, bell peppers, and broccoli are excellent sources of vitamin C.

Vitamin E: Vitamin E is a fat-soluble antioxidant that protects cell membranes from oxidative damage. It works synergistically with vitamin C to enhance its antioxidant effects. Nuts, seeds, vegetable oils, and leafy greens are good sources of vitamin E.

Selenium: Selenium is a trace mineral that acts as an essential component of the antioxidant enzyme glutathione peroxidase. This enzyme helps neutralize free radicals and protect cells from oxidative damage. Selenium can be found in Brazil nuts, seafood, whole grains, and eggs.

Including a variety of foods rich in these antioxidants in the diet can help support cellular health and reduce oxidative stress.

9.3 Phytonutrients as Antioxidants

Phytonutrients, also known as phytochemicals, are natural compounds found in plants that have antioxidant properties. These compounds play a significant role in plant defense against environmental stressors and offer numerous health benefits when consumed by humans.

Different phytonutrients have diverse antioxidant properties and may target specific types of free radicals. Some common phytonutrients with antioxidant activity include:

Flavonoids: Found in fruits, vegetables, and herbs, flavonoids are potent antioxidants that may help reduce the risk of chronic diseases.

Polyphenols: These compounds are abundant in tea, cocoa, berries, and nuts, and have been associated with various health benefits, including heart health and cognitive function.

Carotenoids: Carotenoids are responsible for the vibrant colors in fruits and vegetables. Examples include beta-carotene in carrots, lycopene in tomatoes, and lutein in leafy greens.

Resveratrol: Found in red grapes, berries, and peanuts, resveratrol is known for its potential anti-aging and heart-protective effects.

Curcumin: The active compound in turmeric, curcumin is a powerful antioxidant with anti-inflammatory properties.

By consuming a diverse range of plant-based foods, individuals can benefit from a wide variety of phytonutrients and their antioxidant effects.

9.4 Antioxidant-Rich Foods: Berries, Leafy Greens, and Nuts

Several whole foods are particularly rich in antioxidants and can be easily incorporated into a balanced diet:

Berries: Blueberries, strawberries, raspberries, and blackberries are rich in anthocyanins, flavonoids known for their antioxidant properties.

Leafy Greens: Spinach, kale, Swiss chard, and other leafy greens are excellent sources of vitamins A, C, and E, as well as phytonutrients like lutein and zeaxanthin.

Nuts: Almonds, walnuts, and pistachios are high in vitamin E and other antioxidants, making them a nutritious and antioxidant-rich snack.

Colorful Vegetables: Carrots, sweet potatoes, bell peppers, and tomatoes contain carotenoids with antioxidant properties.

Green Tea: Green tea is rich in catechins, a type of polyphenol with potent antioxidant effects.

Cocoa: Dark chocolate and cocoa powder are rich in flavonoids, particularly flavan

ols, which have been associated with heart health benefits.

By incorporating these antioxidant-rich foods into the diet, individuals can boost their antioxidant intake and support cellular health.

9.5 The Link Between Antioxidants and Aging

Oxidative stress has been linked to the aging process and age-related diseases. As cells are exposed to free radicals over time, cumulative damage can occur to cellular structures, including DNA, proteins, and lipids. This oxidative damage can lead to cellular dysfunction and an increased risk of age-related diseases.

Antioxidants play a crucial role in combating oxidative stress and protecting cells from damage. By neutralizing free radicals, antioxidants help prevent and minimize the harmful effects of oxidative stress on cellular structures.

While antioxidants can't halt the aging process entirely, they can contribute to healthy aging by supporting cellular health and reducing the risk of age-related diseases. A balanced diet rich in antioxidant-containing foods is one of the strategies that may support healthy aging.

9.6 Antioxidants and Immune Function

The immune system plays a vital role in defending the body against pathogens and foreign invaders. Oxidative stress can impair immune function, leaving the body more susceptible to infections and illnesses.

Antioxidants, particularly vitamins C and E, selenium, and zinc, play a critical role in supporting immune function. They help protect immune cells from oxidative damage, ensuring their optimal function.

Vitamin C is involved in the production and function of immune cells, including white blood cells that help fight infections. Vitamin E supports the production of antibodies and enhances the activity of certain immune cells.

Selenium is essential for the function of glutathione peroxidase, an enzyme that helps neutralize free radicals and supports the immune system. Zinc is involved in the development and activation of immune cells.

Consuming a diet rich in antioxidants can help support a robust immune system and protect against infections and illnesses.

9.7 Antioxidants for Skin Health and Radiance

The skin is exposed to various environmental stressors, including ultraviolet (UV) radiation, pollution, and toxins. These stressors can lead to the formation of free radicals, causing oxidative damage to skin cells and contributing to premature aging, wrinkles, and other skin issues.

Antioxidants are essential for maintaining skin health and radiance. They help neutralize free radicals and protect skin cells from oxidative damage.

Vitamin C is a particularly powerful antioxidant for the skin. It supports collagen production, which is essential for skin elasticity and reducing the appearance of wrinkles.

Vitamin E helps protect the skin's lipid barrier, preventing moisture loss and maintaining skin hydration.

Polyphenols and flavonoids found in green tea and certain fruits can also benefit the skin by reducing inflammation and promoting a healthy complexion.

Additionally, beta-carotene and other carotenoids can impart a healthy glow to the skin, as they are associated with a more vibrant complexion.

9.8 Combining Antioxidants for Synergistic Benefits

Antioxidants work synergistically when combined in the diet, enhancing each other's effects and providing optimal protection against oxidative stress.

For example, vitamin C can regenerate vitamin E after it has neutralized a free radical. This regenerative capacity enhances the overall antioxidant capacity of both vitamins.

Additionally, certain phytonutrients can increase the bioavailability and absorption of specific antioxidants. For instance, quercetin, a flavonoid found in apples and onions, has been shown to increase the absorption of vitamin C.

To maximize the benefits of antioxidants, aim to include a variety of antioxidant-rich foods in the diet and consider pairing foods that naturally complement each other's antioxidant properties.

9.9 Cooking Techniques to Preserve Antioxidants in Food

The way food is prepared and cooked can impact the antioxidant content. Some cooking methods can lead to nutrient loss, including antioxidants.

To preserve the antioxidant content in food during cooking:

- Use Short Cooking Times: Brief cooking times at lower temperatures can help retain more antioxidants in vegetables and fruits.

- Avoid Overcooking: Overcooking can cause nutrient loss, including antioxidants. Steaming, sautéing, or stir-frying are better cooking methods to preserve nutrients.

- Store Food Properly: Exposure to air, light, and heat can lead to nutrient degradation. Store fruits and vegetables properly to maintain their antioxidant content.

- Use Minimal Water: Cooking with minimal water can help prevent water-soluble antioxidants from leaching into the cooking water.

While some nutrient loss is inevitable during cooking, adopting cooking methods that retain more antioxidants can help maximize their health benefits.

9.10 Antioxidant Supplements: Benefits and Cautions

While a balanced diet rich in antioxidant-containing foods is the best way to obtain antioxidants, some individuals may consider antioxidant supplements.

Supplements can be beneficial for individuals with specific nutritional deficiencies or those who have difficulty meeting their nutrient needs through diet alone.

However, it is essential to approach antioxidant supplementation with caution, as excessive intake of certain antioxidants can have adverse effects. High doses of vitamin E, for example, may interfere with blood clotting, while excessive beta-carotene intake can lead to a harmless but noticeable yellow-orange discoloration of the skin.

Moreover, antioxidants obtained through whole foods are typically more beneficial than isolated supplements because they work in synergy with other nutrients and compounds present in whole foods.

Consulting with a healthcare professional or registered dietitian before starting any supplementation is essential to determine individual needs and ensure safe and appropriate use.

In conclusion, antioxidants are powerful compounds that play a crucial role in cellular health and overall well-being. By incorporating a variety of antioxidant-rich foods into a balanced diet, individuals can support their immune system, protect against oxidative stress, and promote healthy aging and vibrant skin. Remember that whole foods are the best source of antioxidants, and supplements should be used with caution and under professional guidance.

Chapter 10: Understanding Allergies and Food Intolerances

10.1 Common Food Allergens: Nuts, Dairy, and Shellfish

Food allergies are immune responses triggered by certain proteins in foods. The body's immune system mistakenly identifies these proteins as harmful, leading to the release of histamine and other chemicals that cause allergic reactions.

Some of the most common food allergens include:

Nuts: Peanuts and tree nuts, such as almonds, walnuts, cashews, and pistachios, are common allergens. Allergic reactions to nuts can range from mild symptoms like hives and itching to severe anaphylaxis, a life-threatening reaction.

Dairy: Cow's milk allergy is one of the most prevalent food allergies in infants and young children. It can cause symptoms such as skin rash, gastrointestinal upset, and respiratory issues.

Shellfish: Allergies to shellfish, including shrimp, crab, lobster, and clams, can be severe and often cause immediate allergic reactions.

Other common food allergens include eggs, wheat, soy, fish, and sesame seeds. Food allergies can develop at any age, and even small amounts of allergenic proteins can trigger a reaction in sensitive individuals.

10.2 Gluten Sensitivity and Celiac Disease

Gluten sensitivity and celiac disease are two distinct conditions related to gluten consumption.

Celiac Disease: Celiac disease is an autoimmune disorder triggered by the ingestion of gluten, a protein found in wheat, barley, and rye. In individuals with celiac disease, gluten consumption leads to an immune response that damages the lining of the small intestine. This damage can hinder nutrient absorption and lead to various gastrointestinal and nutritional deficiencies. Symptoms of celiac disease include diarrhea, abdominal pain, bloating, fatigue, and weight loss.

Gluten Sensitivity (Non-Celiac Gluten Sensitivity - NCGS): Gluten sensitivity is a condition in which individuals experience symptoms similar to those of celiac disease, but without the immune system attacking the small intestine. The exact cause of NCGS is not fully understood, but it is not an autoimmune condition like celiac disease. Symptoms of NCGS can include gastrointestinal issues, fatigue, headache, and brain fog.

For individuals with celiac disease or gluten sensitivity, a strict gluten-free diet is essential to manage symptoms and prevent complications.

10.3 Lactose Intolerance and Dairy Alternatives

Lactose intolerance is a common condition characterized by the inability to digest lactose, the sugar found in milk and dairy products, due to a deficiency of the enzyme lactase.

When lactose reaches the large intestine undigested, it can ferment and cause symptoms such as gas, bloating, diarrhea, and abdominal pain.

Individuals with lactose intolerance can manage their condition by avoiding or reducing lactose-containing foods or using lactase supplements to aid digestion.

Dairy Alternatives: There are various dairy alternatives available for individuals with lactose intolerance or those who choose to avoid dairy products. Plant-based milk alternatives, such as almond milk, soy milk, oat milk, and coconut milk, are popular options. These alternatives can provide similar nutrient profiles to cow's milk when fortified.

10.4 Managing Food Allergies in Children

Managing food allergies in children requires a collaborative effort between parents, caregivers, teachers, and healthcare professionals.

Diagnosis: If a child displays symptoms of a food allergy, a comprehensive evaluation by an allergist is essential to diagnose and identify the specific allergens.

Education: Parents and caregivers should receive education on food allergy management, including how to read food labels, recognize symptoms of an allergic reaction, and respond appropriately in case of an emergency.

Safe Environments: It is crucial to create safe environments for children with food allergies, both at home and in school. This may involve implementing allergen-free zones, communicating food allergies to school staff, and providing allergen-free treats for special occasions.

Emergency Plans: Children with severe food allergies should have an emergency action plan, including the administration of epinephrine in case of anaphylaxis.

Education for Peers: Educating classmates and friends about food allergies can promote understanding and empathy, reducing the risk of accidental exposure.

10.5 Food Intolerances vs. Food Allergies

While food allergies and food intolerances can share similar symptoms, they are distinct conditions with different underlying mechanisms.

Food Allergies: Food allergies involve the immune system and are triggered by specific proteins in foods. Symptoms can range from mild to severe and may include skin rashes, itching, hives, swelling, gastrointestinal issues, and anaphylaxis. Allergic reactions occur soon after consuming the allergen and can be life-threatening in some cases.

Food Intolerances: Food intolerances do not involve the immune system and are generally less severe than allergies. They are often caused by the body's inability to properly digest certain components of foods, such as lactose or histamine. Symptoms of food intolerances can include bloating, gas, diarrhea, headaches, and skin issues. Unlike allergies, food intolerances may have a delayed onset of symptoms.

Identifying the specific trigger is crucial for managing food intolerances. This can involve keeping a food diary, undergoing elimination diets, or seeking medical testing.

10.6 The Role of Gut Health in Food Intolerances

The gut plays a central role in food intolerances, as it is responsible for digesting and absorbing nutrients from the foods we eat.

For example, lactose intolerance occurs when the enzyme lactase, which is responsible for breaking down lactose, is deficient. This leads to undigested lactose reaching the large intestine, causing gastrointestinal symptoms.

In some cases, food intolerances can be related to underlying gut issues, such as small intestinal bacterial overgrowth (SIBO) or irritable bowel syndrome (IBS). Addressing these gut-related conditions can help improve food intolerances.

Maintaining a healthy gut through a balanced diet, regular physical activity, stress management, and probiotic-rich foods can support digestive health and reduce the severity of food intolerances.

10.7 Elimination Diets for Identifying Food Triggers

Elimination diets involve removing specific foods or food groups from the diet to identify potential triggers for food allergies or intolerances.

The elimination phase typically lasts for a few weeks to a few months, during which the individual avoids specific foods that are suspected to be causing symptoms. After the elimination phase, foods are gradually reintroduced one at a time, while observing for any symptoms or reactions.

It is essential to conduct an elimination diet under the guidance of a registered dietitian or healthcare professional to ensure that the diet remains balanced and nutritionally adequate.

Food allergies and intolerances can be complex and may involve multiple triggers. Identifying the specific culprits can help individuals modify their diets and manage symptoms effectively.

10.8 Food Allergies and Inflammation

Food allergies, especially when triggered by common allergens like nuts, shellfish, and dairy, can lead to inflammation in the body. The immune system's response to allergenic proteins causes the release of inflammatory mediators, such as histamine and cytokines.

Chronic inflammation can be harmful to overall health and is associated with various chronic diseases, including asthma, eczema, and autoimmune conditions.

Managing food allergies by avoiding allergenic foods can help reduce inflammation and minimize the risk of related health complications.

10.9 Coping with Food Allergies in Social Settings

Managing food allergies in social settings can present challenges, but with proper planning and communication, individuals with food allergies can participate fully in social gatherings

and events.

Communicate: Inform hosts or event organizers about food allergies in advance, so they can accommodate dietary needs.

Bring Safe Snacks: Consider bringing allergen-free snacks or meals to social gatherings to ensure safe food options are available.

Educate Others: Educate friends and family members about food allergies and the importance of avoiding cross-contamination.

Carry Medications: Always carry prescribed medications, such as epinephrine auto-injectors, in case of accidental exposure.

Be Prepared: Have a clear action plan for handling allergic reactions, and inform close friends or family members about the plan.

While social settings can be challenging, being proactive and prepared can help individuals with food allergies enjoy social activities safely.

10.10 Nutritional Considerations for Allergy-Prone Individuals

For individuals with food allergies or intolerances, ensuring a balanced and nutritious diet is essential.

Food Substitutions: Identify suitable substitutions for allergenic foods to ensure nutrient needs are met. For example, if dairy is avoided, calcium-rich plant-based sources can be included in the diet.

Nutrient Supplementation: In some cases, individuals with severe allergies or dietary restrictions may benefit from nutrient supplementation to ensure adequate intake of essential nutrients.

Variety in the Diet: Encourage a diverse diet to obtain a wide range of nutrients from various foods.

Reading Food Labels: Thoroughly read food labels to identify potential allergens or hidden sources of allergenic ingredients.

Consult a Dietitian: Working with a registered dietitian can provide personalized guidance and ensure that nutritional needs are met while managing food allergies or intolerances.

A well-balanced diet, along with proper planning and awareness, can help individuals with food allergies and intolerances lead healthy and fulfilling lives.

Chapter 11: Sports Nutrition for Performance and Recovery

11.1 Macronutrient Ratios for Athletes

For athletes, proper macronutrient intake is essential to support energy levels, optimize performance, and facilitate recovery. The ideal macronutrient ratio can vary depending on the type of sport, training intensity, and individual goals. However, some general guidelines can be helpful:

Carbohydrates: Carbohydrates are the primary source of energy for athletes, especially during high-intensity activities. Aim to include complex carbohydrates from whole grains, fruits, and vegetables in the diet to provide sustained energy.

Proteins: Protein is crucial for muscle repair and growth, making it vital for athletes to support recovery. Include lean sources of protein such as poultry, fish, tofu, beans, and dairy products in the diet.

Fats: Healthy fats are essential for hormone production and joint health. Opt for sources like avocados, nuts, seeds, and olive oil.

The specific macronutrient ratio for athletes can vary based on training goals, body composition, and individual preferences. Consulting with a sports dietitian can help determine the ideal macronutrient distribution to optimize athletic performance.

11.2 Pre- and Post-Workout Nutrition

Pre- and post-workout nutrition plays a critical role in athletic performance and recovery.

Pre-Workout Nutrition: The goal of pre-workout nutrition is to provide the body with the necessary fuel to perform optimally during exercise. The meal or snack consumed before a workout should be easily digestible and rich in carbohydrates for readily available energy. Including a small amount of protein can also help with muscle support during exercise. Some suitable pre-workout snacks include a banana with almond butter, a whole-grain sandwich with lean protein, or a smoothie with fruits and yogurt.

Post-Workout Nutrition: After exercise, the body requires nutrients to replenish glycogen stores, repair muscle tissue, and promote recovery. Consuming a combination of carbohydrates and protein within the first hour after exercise is beneficial. This can be achieved through a protein shake, a balanced meal with lean protein and complex carbohydrates, or a sports recovery drink.

Timing is crucial for pre- and post-workout nutrition. Consuming a meal or snack about 1-2 hours before exercise allows for proper digestion, while post-workout nutrition should be consumed as soon as possible to optimize recovery.

11.3 Hydration Strategies for Active Individuals

Staying properly hydrated is essential for athletes to maintain performance and prevent dehydration.

Hydration Before Exercise: Start workouts well-hydrated by consuming fluids throughout the day before exercise. Aim to drink water, herbal teas, or diluted fruit juices to maintain hydration.

Hydration During Exercise: During exercise, sip water regularly to replace fluids lost through sweat. The exact fluid needs vary depending on factors such as exercise intensity, duration, and environmental conditions. Electrolyte drinks may be beneficial for activities lasting longer than one hour or in hot weather to replenish sodium and other electrolytes lost in sweat.

Hydration After Exercise: After exercise, continue to hydrate to restore fluid balance and support recovery. Drinking water or a recovery beverage with electrolytes can be beneficial.

Monitoring Hydration: Pay attention to signs of dehydration, such as dark urine, fatigue, dizziness, and dry mouth. Monitoring body weight before and after exercise can also help estimate fluid loss.

Hydration needs can vary among athletes, so it's essential to individualize fluid intake based on personal factors and exercise demands.

11.4 Electrolyte Balance during Exercise

Electrolytes are minerals that carry electrical charges and play a crucial role in maintaining proper fluid balance, nerve function, and muscle contractions.

During exercise, electrolytes, particularly sodium, potassium, and magnesium, are lost through sweat. Replenishing these electrolytes is crucial to prevent dehydration and maintain performance.

Electrolyte-rich foods and beverages can help maintain electrolyte balance:

Sodium: Foods like pretzels, pickles, and sports drinks can help replace lost sodium.

Potassium: Bananas, oranges, and potatoes are excellent sources of potassium.

Magnesium: Nuts, seeds, leafy greens, and whole grains are good sources of magnesium.

For prolonged or intense exercise lasting over an hour, consuming electrolyte drinks or gels during activity can help maintain electrolyte balance.

11.5 Protein Timing for Muscle Synthesis

Protein is crucial for muscle repair and growth, making its timing essential for athletes to optimize recovery and performance.

Pre-Workout Protein: Consuming a small amount of protein before exercise can support muscle protein synthesis during the workout. A whey protein shake or a protein-rich snack, such as Greek yogurt or a protein bar, can be beneficial.

Post-Workout Protein: The most critical time for protein intake is within the first hour after exercise. Consuming a protein-rich meal or shake during this window helps promote muscle repair and recovery. Whey protein is often recommended for its rapid absorption, but other protein sources like lean meats, dairy products, and plant-based proteins can also be effective.

Additionally, spreading protein intake throughout the day, including at regular meals and snacks, can support muscle synthesis and recovery over time.

11.6 Carbohydrate Loading for Endurance Activities

Carbohydrate loading, also known as glycogen loading, is a strategy used by endurance athletes to maximize glycogen stores in the muscles and liver before long-duration events.

Carbohydrate loading typically involves:

Tapering Training: Reducing training intensity and volume in the days leading up to the event to allow the muscles to store more glycogen.

Increasing Carbohydrate Intake: Gradually increasing carbohydrate intake in the days leading up to the event to saturate glycogen stores.

Common carbohydrate-rich foods used for loading include pasta, rice, potatoes, bread, and fruits.

Carbohydrate loading is most beneficial for endurance events lasting longer than 90 minutes, such as marathons, triathlons, and long-distance cycling races.

11.7 Supplements for Athletic Performance

While a well-balanced diet can provide most of the nutrients athletes need, some supplements may be beneficial for specific situations:

Creatine: Creatine is a popular supplement for athletes engaged in high-intensity, short-duration activities. It can improve performance in activities like weightlifting and sprinting.

Caffeine: Caffeine can enhance endurance performance by increasing alertness and reducing perceived effort during exercise.

Beta-Alanine: Beta-alanine may improve high-intensity exercise performance and delay fatigue.

Branch-Chain Amino Acids (BCAAs): BCAAs can support muscle recovery and reduce muscle soreness.

Iron: Iron supplements may be necessary for athletes, especially female athletes, who have low iron levels.

Supplements should be used with caution and under the guidance of a sports dietitian or healthcare professional to ensure safety and effectiveness.

11.8 Nutrition Strategies for Different Sports

Different sports have varying energy demands and nutrient requirements. Tailoring nutrition strategies to specific sports can optimize athletic performance.

Endurance Sports (Running, Cycling, Triathlon): Endurance athletes require a higher intake of carbohydrates to sustain prolonged efforts.

Carbohydrate loading before long events and carbohydrate-rich snacks during activity are crucial.

Strength and Power Sports (Weightlifting, Sprinting): Athletes in these sports benefit from protein-rich diets to support muscle repair and growth. Adequate hydration is also essential.

Team Sports (Soccer, Basketball, Hockey): Team sport athletes need a balanced diet to support overall performance and recovery. Carbohydrates for energy, protein for muscle support,

and fats for endurance are all essential.

11.9 Overcoming Nutritional Challenges in Training

Athletes may face various nutritional challenges during training, such as travel, limited food options, and time constraints. To overcome these challenges:

Plan Ahead: Plan meals and snacks in advance, especially during travel or busy training schedules.

Pack Snacks: Bring portable and nutritious snacks like nuts, seeds, energy bars, and fruits to maintain energy levels.

Hydrate Smartly: Carry a water bottle to stay hydrated throughout the day.

Fuel During Training: Practice fueling during training sessions to identify what works best for individual needs.

11.10 Recovery Foods and Techniques for Athletes

Recovery is a critical aspect of athletic training to support muscle repair and reduce the risk of injury.

Recovery Foods: Consuming a meal or snack with carbohydrates and protein within an hour after exercise can support muscle recovery and glycogen replenishment. Chocolate milk, smoothies with fruits and protein, or a balanced meal with lean protein and whole grains are suitable recovery options.

Rest and Sleep: Proper rest and sleep are essential for recovery. Aim for 7-9 hours of quality sleep per night.

Active Recovery: Light exercise, such as gentle stretching or walking, can help promote blood flow and reduce muscle stiffness after intense training.

Compression Garments: Wearing compression garments may aid in reducing muscle soreness and promoting recovery.

Hydration: Rehydrate with water and electrolyte-rich beverages after exercise to restore fluid balance.

Overall, proper nutrition and recovery strategies are essential for athletes to maximize performance, support overall health, and reduce the risk of injuries. Individualized nutrition plans and consulting with sports dietitians can help athletes optimize their dietary choices for their specific needs and goals.

Chapter 12: Nutrition for a Healthy Heart

12.1 Understanding Cardiovascular Health

Cardiovascular health refers to the well-being of the heart and blood vessels, encompassing various aspects of heart function and overall circulatory system health. A healthy cardiovascular system is crucial for optimal blood circulation, nutrient delivery, waste removal, and oxygen transport to all organs and tissues in the body.

Factors that impact cardiovascular health include diet, physical activity, smoking, stress, and genetics. Leading a heart-healthy lifestyle can reduce the risk of cardiovascular diseases such as heart attacks, strokes, and hypertension.

12.2 The Impact of Diet on Heart Health

Diet plays a significant role in heart health, and making smart dietary choices can promote cardiovascular well-being. Some key dietary factors for heart health include:

Balanced Diet: Consume a balanced diet that includes a variety of fruits, vegetables, whole grains, lean proteins, and healthy fats. Avoid excessive intake of processed and high-sugar foods.

Portion Control: Pay attention to portion sizes to avoid overeating and excess calorie intake, which can contribute to weight gain and heart health issues.

Limiting Saturated and Trans Fats: Reduce the intake of saturated and trans fats found in fried foods, processed snacks, and certain types of meat. These fats can raise LDL cholesterol levels, increasing the risk of heart disease.

Incorporating Heart-Healthy Fats: Include sources of heart-healthy fats such as avocados, nuts, seeds, and olive oil, which can help improve cholesterol levels and reduce inflammation.

12.3 Heart-Healthy Fats: Omega-3 and Monounsaturated Fats

Omega-3 fatty acids and monounsaturated fats are beneficial for heart health due to their positive effects on blood lipid levels, inflammation, and blood vessel function.

Omega-3 Fatty Acids: Found in fatty fish like salmon, mackerel, and sardines, as well as chia seeds, flaxseeds, and walnuts, omega-3 fatty acids have been shown to lower triglycerides, reduce blood pressure, and improve heart rhythm.

Monounsaturated Fats: Found in olive oil, avocados, nuts, and seeds, monounsaturated fats can help lower LDL cholesterol levels while maintaining or increasing HDL cholesterol levels, promoting heart health.

Including these heart-healthy fats in the diet while reducing saturated and trans fat intake can contribute to a healthier cardiovascular system.

12.4 Sodium Reduction for Blood Pressure Management

High sodium intake has been linked to hypertension (high blood pressure), which is a significant risk factor for heart disease and stroke.

Reducing sodium intake can help manage blood pressure levels. Some strategies for sodium reduction include:

Reading Labels: Check food labels for sodium content and choose lower-sodium options.

Limiting Processed Foods: Processed foods, such as canned soups, frozen meals, and salty snacks, are often high in sodium. Opt for fresh or minimally processed foods instead.

Using Herbs and Spices: Flavor foods with herbs, spices, and other salt-free seasonings instead of relying on salt for taste.

Cooking at Home: Preparing meals at home allows better control over sodium content.

Gradual Reduction: Gradually reduce sodium intake to allow taste buds to adjust to lower sodium levels.

12.5 Fiber and Cholesterol Levels

Fiber is beneficial for heart health, particularly in its role in managing cholesterol levels.

Soluble fiber, found in oats, beans, lentils, fruits, and vegetables, can help reduce LDL cholesterol levels. It binds to cholesterol in the digestive tract, preventing its absorption into the bloodstream.

Including fiber-rich foods in the diet can be an effective strategy for managing cholesterol levels and reducing the risk of heart disease.

12.6 Antioxidants for Reducing Oxidative Stress in Blood Vessels

Oxidative stress, caused by an imbalance between free radicals and antioxidants in the body, can damage blood vessels and contribute to cardiovascular disease.

Antioxidants, such as vitamins A, C, and E, as well as polyphenols found in fruits, vegetables, and nuts, help neutralize free radicals and reduce oxidative stress.

Consuming a diet rich in antioxidant-containing foods can support cardiovascular health and reduce the risk of atherosclerosis and other heart-related conditions.

12.7 Plant-Based Diets and Cardiovascular Health

Plant-based diets, such as vegetarian and vegan diets, have been associated with improved heart health due to their focus on nutrient-dense plant foods and reduced intake of saturated fat and cholesterol.

Plant-based diets have been shown to lower LDL cholesterol levels, blood pressure, and the risk of heart disease.

Including a variety of plant foods like whole grains, legumes, fruits, vegetables, nuts, and seeds can support heart health and overall well-being.

12.8 The Role of Exercise in Cardiovascular Fitness

Regular physical activity and exercise are essential for maintaining cardiovascular fitness and reducing the risk of heart disease.

Exercise benefits the heart in several ways:

Improving Heart Strength: Regular exercise strengthens the heart muscle, allowing it to pump blood more efficiently.

Lowering Blood Pressure: Exercise can help reduce blood pressure, a significant risk factor for heart disease.

Improving Cholesterol Levels: Physical activity can raise HDL (good) cholesterol levels and lower LDL (bad) cholesterol levels.

Enhancing Circulation: Exercise improves blood flow and circulation, delivering oxygen and nutrients to all body tissues.

Reducing Inflammation: Regular exercise can reduce systemic inflammation, which is linked to heart disease.

Aim for at least 150 minutes of moderate-intensity exercise or 75 minutes of vigorous-intensity exercise per week to support cardiovascular fitness.

12.9 Nutritional Considerations for Hypertension and Cholesterol

Individuals with hypertension (high blood pressure) or high cholesterol levels may need specific dietary considerations to manage these conditions and promote heart health.

Hypertension: A heart-healthy diet for hypertension should focus on reducing sodium intake, increasing potassium-rich foods, such as fruits and vegetables, and maintaining a balanced diet to support weight management.

High Cholesterol: To manage high cholesterol levels, a diet low in saturated and trans fats is essential. Including soluble fiber from oats, legumes, and fruits can help lower LDL cholesterol levels. Foods containing omega-3 fatty acids and monounsaturated fats can also contribute to better cholesterol profiles.

Working with a healthcare provider or a registered dietitian can provide personalized nutrition guidance for managing hypertension and cholesterol.

12.10 Lifestyle Habits for a Strong and Healthy Heart

Beyond nutrition, other lifestyle habits play a crucial role in maintaining a strong and healthy heart:

Maintaining a Healthy Weight: Achieving and maintaining a healthy weight can reduce the risk of heart disease and other chronic conditions.

Avoiding Smoking: Smoking is a significant risk factor for heart disease. Quitting smoking can have immediate and long-term benefits for heart health.

Managing Stress: Chronic stress can impact heart health. Adopting stress management techniques such as meditation, yoga, or mindfulness can be beneficial.

Getting Adequate Sleep: Poor sleep quality or insufficient sleep can increase the risk of heart disease. Aim for 7-9 hours of quality sleep each night.

Limiting Alcohol: Excessive alcohol consumption can negatively affect heart health. If you drink, do so in moderation as per recommended guidelines.

Regular Checkups: Regular medical checkups can help monitor and manage cardiovascular risk factors.

Incorporating these lifestyle habits alongside a heart-healthy diet can contribute to overall cardiovascular well-being and support a strong and healthy heart.

Chapter 13: Nutrition during Pregnancy and Lactation

Pregnancy is a crucial time for the health and development of both the mother and the growing fetus. Proper nutrition during pregnancy and lactation is essential to support the increased nutrient demands, promote optimal fetal development, and ensure the well-being of the mother.

13.1 Nutritional Needs during Pregnancy

During pregnancy, the body's nutrient requirements increase to support the growing baby and changes in the mother's body. Key nutrients to focus on during pregnancy include:

Folic Acid: Important for preventing neural tube defects, folic acid is vital during the early stages of pregnancy. It can be found in leafy greens, fortified cereals, and legumes.

Iron: Iron is necessary for red blood cell production and preventing iron-deficiency anemia during pregnancy. Good sources include lean meats, beans, tofu, and fortified cereals.

Calcium: Essential for fetal bone development, calcium can be obtained from dairy products, fortified plant-based milk, and leafy greens.

Protein: Protein is crucial for the growth and development of the baby. Good sources include lean meats, poultry, fish, eggs, legumes, and dairy products.

Omega-3 Fatty Acids: Important for brain and eye development, omega-3 fatty acids are found in fatty fish, chia seeds, flaxseeds, and walnuts.

Vitamin D: Vital for calcium absorption, vitamin D can be obtained from sunlight exposure and fortified foods.

Iodine: Essential for thyroid function and fetal brain development, iodine can be found in iodized salt and seafood.

Meeting these increased nutrient needs is critical for the health and well-being of both the mother and the baby.

13.2 The Importance of Folate for Fetal Development

Folate, also known as folic acid when in its synthetic form, is a B-vitamin that plays a crucial role in fetal development, particularly during the early stages of pregnancy.

Folate is essential for proper neural tube formation, which occurs within the first 28 days of pregnancy when many women may not yet know they are pregnant. Adequate folate intake can help prevent neural tube defects such as spina bifida.

To ensure sufficient folate intake during pregnancy, women are advised to take a prenatal vitamin with folic acid, in addition to consuming folate-rich foods like leafy greens, legumes, fortified cereals, and citrus fruits.

13.3 Iron and Calcium Requirements during Pregnancy

Iron and calcium are two essential minerals during pregnancy.

Iron: Iron is necessary for the production of red blood cells, which transport oxygen to the baby and the mother's body. Pregnant women may experience increased iron needs due to the expansion of blood volume. Iron-rich foods like lean meats, beans, tofu, and fortified cereals should be included in the diet, and iron supplements may be prescribed if needed.

Calcium: Calcium is crucial for fetal bone development, as the baby's skeleton is formed during pregnancy. Pregnant women need to ensure sufficient calcium intake from sources such as dairy products, fortified plant-based milk, and leafy greens.

A balanced diet that includes a variety of nutrient-dense foods can help meet these increased iron and calcium needs during pregnancy.

13.4 Managing Nausea and Food Aversions

Many pregnant women experience nausea and food aversions, especially during the first trimester. To manage these symptoms:

Eat Small, Frequent Meals: Consuming smaller, more frequent meals can help manage nausea and prevent an empty stomach.

Avoid Triggers: Identify and avoid foods or smells that trigger nausea.

Stay Hydrated: Drink fluids regularly to prevent dehydration.

Ginger: Ginger, in the form of tea or ginger candies, can help ease nausea for some women.

Bland Foods: Opt for bland, easy-to-digest foods like crackers, rice, and bananas.

Prenatal vitamins can help fill nutrient gaps caused by food aversions, but it's essential to discuss any symptoms with a healthcare provider for proper guidance.

13.5 Gestational Diabetes and Nutrition

Gestational diabetes is a form of diabetes that occurs during pregnancy. It can impact both the mother and the baby's health.

Managing gestational diabetes typically involves:

Balanced Diet: A balanced diet with controlled carbohydrate intake can help stabilize blood sugar levels.

Monitoring Blood Sugar: Regularly monitoring blood glucose levels helps manage gestational diabetes effectively.

Physical Activity: Regular physical activity can support blood sugar control.

Working closely with a healthcare provider and a registered dietitian is crucial for managing gestational diabetes and promoting a healthy pregnancy.

13.6 Foods to Avoid during Pregnancy

During pregnancy, certain foods should be avoided or limited to reduce the risk of foodborne illnesses and other potential risks to the baby. These include:

Raw or Undercooked Meats: These can contain harmful bacteria.

Unpasteurized Dairy Products: Raw milk and certain soft cheeses can carry harmful bacteria.

Raw Seafood: Sushi and other raw seafood should be avoided due to potential contaminants.

High-Mercury Fish: Large fish like swordfish, shark, and king mackerel may contain high levels of mercury.

Alcohol: Alcohol consumption during pregnancy is associated with developmental issues and should be avoided.

Caffeine: Limiting caffeine intake to moderate levels is recommended.

It's essential to follow food safety guidelines and discuss any dietary concerns with a healthcare provider during pregnancy.

13.7 Nutrition for Breastfeeding Mothers

Nutrition is crucial during lactation to support the production of breast milk and provide the necessary nutrients for the baby.

Caloric Needs: Breastfeeding mothers need extra calories to produce milk, but the exact amount varies depending on individual factors.

Hydration: Staying well-hydrated is essential for milk production.

Nutrient-Dense Diet: A balanced diet with a variety of nutrient-dense foods supports both the mother and the baby.

Omega-3 Fatty Acids: Including sources of omega-3 fatty acids in the diet can benefit the baby's brain development.

Avoiding Certain Foods: Some babies may be sensitive to specific foods in the mother's diet. If the baby shows signs of discomfort or allergies, the mother may need to adjust her diet.

Prenatal vitamins are often recommended during lactation to ensure nutrient needs are met.

13.8 Postpartum Nutrition and Recovery

After childbirth, nutrition remains essential for postpartum recovery and supporting the mother's health.

A well-balanced diet with nutrient-dense foods, including whole grains, lean proteins, fruits, vegetables, and healthy fats, can help support healing and energy levels.

Adequate hydration is crucial during postpartum recovery, especially for breastfeeding mothers.

Mothers should avoid restrictive diets during this time and focus on nourishing their bodies to promote healing and well-being.

13.9 Meeting Nutritional Needs for Twins and Multiples

Carrying twins or multiples can increase the nutritional demands during pregnancy.

Nutrient Intake: Women pregnant with multiples may need higher calorie and protein intake to support the growth of multiple babies.

Prenatal Vitamins: Prenatal vitamins with adequate folic acid, iron, and other essential nutrients are vital during this time.

Consultation: Working with a healthcare provider and a registered dietitian can help ensure proper nutrient intake for a healthy pregnancy.

13.10 Healthy Weight Management during and after Pregnancy

Maintaining a healthy weight during and after pregnancy is essential for the mother's well-being and the baby's health.

Pregnancy Weight Gain: Weight gain recommendations during pregnancy vary based on pre-pregnancy weight and the number of babies carried.

Postpartum Weight Loss

: Slow and steady weight loss is generally recommended after childbirth. Focusing on a balanced diet and regular physical activity can aid in gradual weight loss.

Breastfeeding and Weight Loss: Breastfeeding can support postpartum weight loss in some women.

Avoid Crash Diets: Crash diets are not recommended during pregnancy or postpartum, as they may compromise nutrient intake and affect milk supply in breastfeeding mothers.

Overall, adopting healthy lifestyle habits, following a balanced diet, and seeking support from healthcare providers and dietitians are essential during and after pregnancy to promote both maternal and infant   health.

Chapter 14: Nutrition for Healthy Aging

As individuals age, their nutritional needs change, and adopting a healthy and balanced diet becomes even more crucial for promoting overall health and well-being. Proper nutrition can support healthy aging by providing essential nutrients to maintain muscle mass, bone health, brain function, and cellular health while managing chronic conditions. In this chapter, we will explore the key nutritional considerations for healthy aging and building habits that contribute to a fulfilling senior life.

14.1 The Aging Process and Nutritional Needs

Aging is a natural process that brings about changes in the body's metabolism and nutrient requirements. Some common age-related changes include a decrease in muscle mass and bone density, changes in taste and smell perception, reduced absorption of certain nutrients, and altered metabolism.

As individuals age, it becomes important to:

Consume Nutrient-Dense Foods: Choose foods that are rich in essential nutrients and provide the most nutrition per calorie.

Stay Hydrated: Proper hydration is essential for older adults to support overall health and prevent dehydration.

Balance Caloric Intake: Adjust caloric intake to match changes in metabolism and activity levels to prevent weight gain or loss.

14.2 Maintaining Muscle Mass and Strength

Maintaining muscle mass and strength is critical for healthy aging, as it supports mobility, balance, and overall functionality. Some key strategies to promote muscle health include:

Protein Intake: Consuming an adequate amount of protein is essential for muscle maintenance and repair. Protein sources can include lean meats, poultry, fish, legumes, and dairy products.

Strength Training: Engaging in regular strength training exercises can help preserve muscle mass and enhance strength.

Balanced Diet: A balanced diet that includes a variety of nutrients can support overall muscle health.

14.3 Nutrients for Bone Health: Calcium and Vitamin D

Bone health becomes increasingly important with age, as bones naturally become more fragile. Calcium and vitamin D are essential nutrients for maintaining strong and healthy bones:

Calcium: Calcium-rich foods, such as dairy products, leafy greens, and fortified plant-based milk, should be included in the diet to support bone health.

Vitamin D: Vitamin D, obtained from sunlight exposure and fortified foods, aids in calcium absorption and is crucial for bone health.

Supplements: Some older adults may require calcium and vitamin D supplements, but this should be determined based on individual needs and blood tests.

14.4 Antioxidants and Cellular Health

Antioxidants play a vital role in reducing oxidative stress and protecting cells from damage caused by free radicals. Including antioxidant-rich foods in the diet can promote cellular health and reduce the risk of chronic diseases:

Vitamin A: Found in carrots, sweet potatoes, and leafy greens, vitamin A supports vision and immune function.

Vitamin C: Abundant in citrus fruits, strawberries, and bell peppers, vitamin C supports the immune system and collagen production.

Vitamin E: Found in nuts, seeds, and vegetable oils, vitamin E protects cells from oxidative damage.

Flavonoids: These plant compounds found in berries, tea, and cocoa have antioxidant properties.

14.5 Brain-Boosting Foods: Omega-3 Fatty Acids and Antioxidants

As people age, maintaining brain health and cognitive function becomes a priority. Certain nutrients have been associated with brain health:

Omega-3 Fatty Acids: Found in fatty fish, chia seeds, flaxseeds, and walnuts, omega-3 fatty acids support brain function and reduce inflammation.

Antioxidants: As previously mentioned, antioxidants can protect brain cells from oxidative damage.

B Vitamins: B vitamins, especially vitamin B12, found in animal products and fortified plant-based foods, are crucial for brain health.

Including these brain-boosting nutrients in the diet can contribute to better cognitive function and brain health.

14.6 Managing Chronic Conditions through Diet

Many older adults live with chronic conditions such as hypertension, diabetes, and heart disease. Dietary choices can play a significant role in managing these conditions:

Hypertension: Reducing sodium intake, increasing potassium-rich foods, and adopting the DASH (Dietary Approaches to Stop Hypertension) diet can help manage blood pressure.

Diabetes: Carbohydrate control, portion management, and choosing foods with a low glycemic index can aid in blood sugar management.

Heart Disease: Adopting a heart-healthy diet low in saturated and trans fats, sodium, and cholesterol can support heart health.

Individuals with chronic conditions should work closely with healthcare providers and registered dietitians to develop personalized dietary plans.

14.7 Hydration and Aging

Proper hydration is essential for older adults to maintain overall health and well-being. Dehydration can be more common in older adults due to reduced thirst perception and changes in kidney function.

To stay hydrated:

Drink Fluids Regularly: Even if not feeling thirsty, older adults should drink fluids throughout the day.

Monitor Fluid Intake: Keeping track of fluid intake can help ensure adequate hydration.

Include Water-Rich Foods: Fruits, vegetables, soups, and herbal teas can contribute to overall hydration.

14.8 Superfoods for Longevity and Vitality

While there is no single food that guarantees longevity, some nutrient-dense foods have been associated with better health outcomes in older adults:

Berries: Blueberries, strawberries, and other berries are rich in antioxidants and have been linked to improved cognitive function.

Leafy Greens: Spinach, kale, and other leafy greens are excellent sources of vitamins, minerals, and antioxidants.

Nuts and Seeds: Almonds, chia seeds, and walnuts are packed with healthy fats, protein, and vitamins.

Fish: Fatty fish like salmon and sardines provide omega-3 fatty acids for brain and heart health.

Including these superfoods in the diet can contribute to overall vitality and well-being in older adults.

14.9 The Role of Protein in Elderly Nutrition

Protein becomes even more critical in older adults to support muscle health, immune function, and wound healing. Adequate protein intake can help prevent muscle loss and promote overall health.

Protein sources can include:

Lean Meats: Chicken, turkey, and lean cuts of beef or pork provide high-quality protein.

Fish: Fatty fish like salmon also provide omega-3 fatty acids.

Legumes: Beans, lentils, and chickpeas are excellent plant-based sources of protein.

Dairy Products: Yogurt, milk, and cheese are good sources of protein and calcium.

For older adults with decreased appetite or difficulty consuming protein-rich foods, protein supplements may be considered under the guidance of healthcare providers.

14.10 Building Healthy Habits for a Fulfilling Senior Life

Promoting a fulfilling senior life involves adopting healthy habits that support physical, mental, and emotional well-being:

Physical Activity: Engaging in regular physical activity can support cardiovascular health, muscle strength, and mental well-being.

Social Connections: Maintaining social connections can reduce feelings of isolation and support emotional health.

Mental Stimulation: Engaging in mentally stimulating activities, such as puzzles, reading, or learning new skills, can support cognitive function.

Balanced Diet: A balanced diet that includes a variety of nutrient-dense foods can support overall health and vitality.

Regular Checkups: Regular medical checkups can help monitor health status and identify any potential issues early on.

Aging is a natural part of life, and maintaining a healthy lifestyle, including proper nutrition and regular physical activity, can contribute to a fulfilling and vibrant senior life. Seeking support from healthcare providers and registered dietitians can help older adults develop personalized strategies for healthy aging.

Chapter 15: Nutrition for Immune Support

The immune system plays a critical role in protecting the body from harmful pathogens and maintaining overall health. Proper nutrition is essential for supporting immune function and enhancing the body's ability to defend against infections and diseases. In this chapter, we will explore the key nutrients and lifestyle factors that contribute to a robust immune system and how to create an immune-supportive meal plan.

15.1 The Immune System and Its Functions

The immune system is a complex network of cells, tissues, and organs that work together to defend the body against harmful invaders, such as bacteria, viruses, and toxins. It plays a crucial role in maintaining health and preventing infections. The immune system functions through various mechanisms, including:

Innate Immune Response: The first line of defense that provides immediate protection against pathogens.

Adaptive Immune Response: A specific and targeted response that develops over time after exposure to a pathogen.

The immune system relies on a range of nutrients and lifestyle factors to function optimally and protect the body.

15.2 Nutrients for Immune Health: Vitamins A, C, D, and Zinc

Several key nutrients are essential for supporting immune health:

Vitamin A: Important for maintaining the integrity of the skin and mucous membranes, which act as physical barriers against pathogens. Good sources of vitamin A include carrots, sweet potatoes, and leafy greens.

Vitamin C: A powerful antioxidant that helps boost the production of white blood cells and supports immune function. Citrus fruits, strawberries, and bell peppers are rich sources of vitamin C.

Vitamin D: Plays a crucial role in regulating immune function and reducing inflammation. Sunlight exposure and fortified foods can provide vitamin D.

Zinc: Necessary for the normal development and function of immune cells. Zinc can be found in foods like oysters, beef, and pumpkin seeds.

Including foods rich in these nutrients can help support a robust immune system.

15.3 Probiotics and Gut Health in Immune Function

A significant portion of the immune system resides in the gut. Probiotics, which are beneficial bacteria, play a crucial role in maintaining gut health and supporting immune function.

Fermented Foods: Yogurt, kefir, sauerkraut, and kimchi are excellent sources of probiotics.

Prebiotic Foods: Foods high in prebiotic fibers, such as onions, garlic, and bananas, can help feed beneficial gut bacteria.

Maintaining a healthy balance of gut bacteria through probiotics and prebiotics can support immune health.

15.4 Hydration and Immune Response

Proper hydration is essential for maintaining optimal immune function. Water helps transport immune cells and nutrients throughout the body and supports the elimination of waste products.

Staying Hydrated: Drinking enough water and consuming hydrating foods like fruits and vegetables can help maintain proper hydration.

Limiting Dehydrating Substances: Reducing the intake of dehydrating substances like alcohol and caffeine can support hydration.

Adequate hydration is crucial for a well-functioning immune system.

15.5 Anti-Inflammatory Foods for Immune Support

Chronic inflammation can weaken the immune system and contribute to various health issues. Consuming anti-inflammatory foods can help reduce inflammation and support immune health.

Omega-3 Fatty Acids: Found in fatty fish, flaxseeds, and chia seeds, omega-3 fatty acids have anti-inflammatory properties.

Turmeric: Contains the compound curcumin, which has potent anti-inflammatory effects.

Berries: Rich in antioxidants, berries can help combat inflammation.

By incorporating these anti-inflammatory foods into the diet, individuals can support a healthy immune response.

15.6 The Connection Between Stress and Immunity

Chronic stress can negatively impact immune function. The release of stress hormones can suppress the immune system, making the body more susceptible to infections.

Stress Management Techniques: Practicing stress-reduction techniques like meditation, deep breathing, and yoga can support immune health.

Physical Activity: Regular exercise can help reduce stress and support immune function.

Prioritizing self-care and stress management is vital for maintaining a strong immune system.

15.7 Immune-Boosting Foods: Garlic, Ginger, and Turmeric

Certain foods have been traditionally known for their immune-boosting properties:

Garlic: Contains compounds that have antiviral and antibacterial properties.

Ginger: Has anti-inflammatory effects and supports immune function.

Turmeric: Contains curcumin, which has immune-enhancing properties.

Incorporating these immune-boosting foods into the diet can provide additional support for the immune system.

15.8 Exercise and Its Impact on Immune Function

Regular physical activity has numerous benefits for overall health, including immune function:

Enhanced Immune Response: Exercise can stimulate immune cells, enhancing the body's ability to fight off infections.

Reduced Inflammation: Regular exercise can help reduce chronic inflammation.

Moderate Exercise: Engaging in moderate-intensity exercise is recommended for immune support, as excessive exercise may have the opposite effect.

15.9 Immune Support for Older Adults

As individuals age, their immune system may weaken, making them more vulnerable to infections. Older adults can support their immune health through:

Nutritious Diet: Consuming a well-balanced diet with immune-supportive nutrients is crucial.

Vaccinations: Keeping up with recommended vaccinations can protect against preventable illnesses.

Regular Physical Activity: Exercise can help maintain immune function in older adults.

Regular Checkups: Regular medical checkups can help monitor health and address any concerns promptly.

15.10 Creating an Immune-Supportive Meal Plan

Designing a meal plan that supports immune health involves incorporating a variety of nutrient-dense foods:

Fruits and Vegetables: Rich in vitamins and antioxidants, fruits and vegetables should be a staple in the diet.

Lean Proteins: Including sources of lean proteins like poultry, fish, legumes, and tofu can support immune function.

Whole Grains: Opting for whole grains like brown rice, quinoa, and whole-wheat bread provides essential nutrients.

Healthy Fats: Incorporating sources of healthy fats like avocados, nuts, and olive oil can help reduce inflammation.

Probiotic Foods: Including fermented foods like yogurt and kefir supports gut health.

Hydration: Staying well-hydrated with water and hydrating foods is crucial for immune function.

Creating a balanced meal plan that includes a variety of immune-supportive foods can promote overall health and well-being.

Conclusion:

Maintaining a strong and healthy immune system is essential for protecting the body from infections and promoting overall well-being. Proper nutrition, hydration, and lifestyle habits play a crucial role in supporting immune function. By incorporating immune-boosting nutrients, probiotics, anti-inflammatory foods, and stress management techniques into the diet, individuals can optimize their immune health. Regular exercise, vaccinations, and regular checkups also contribute to a well-functioning immune system. By adopting an immune-supportive meal plan and making lifestyle changes, individuals can enhance their ability to fight off infections and lead a healthy, vibrant life.

Chapter 16: Nutrition for Mental Well-Being

In recent years, research has highlighted the powerful link between nutrition and mental well-being. The foods we consume not only affect our physical health but also play a significant role in shaping our cognitive function, mood, and emotional well-being. This chapter delves into the intricate relationship between nutrition and mental health, exploring how specific nutrients and dietary patterns can positively impact our cognitive function and emotional state.

16.1 The Gut-Brain Connection

The gut-brain connection refers to the bidirectional communication between the gastrointestinal system and the brain. This connection is facilitated by the enteric nervous system (ENS), often called the "second brain," which lines the digestive tract and contains millions of neurons. The ENS communicates with the central nervous system (CNS), influencing emotions, mood, and even cognitive processes.

The gut microbiota, a vast and diverse community of microorganisms residing in the gut, also plays a crucial role in the gut-brain connection. These microbes produce various neuroactive compounds, including neurotransmitters like serotonin and gamma-aminobutyric acid (GABA), which can influence mood and emotional well-being.

Consuming a diet rich in fiber, prebiotics, and probiotics can promote a healthy gut microbiota, leading to improved mood and mental health.

16.2 Foods that Support Cognitive Function

Certain foods have been shown to support cognitive function and enhance brain health. These foods contain compounds that promote neuronal growth, protect brain cells from damage, and improve cognitive performance.

Blueberries: Rich in antioxidants called flavonoids, blueberries have been associated with improved memory and cognitive function.

Turmeric: The active compound curcumin in turmeric has anti-inflammatory and antioxidant properties, which may benefit brain health.

Nuts and Seeds: These are excellent sources of healthy fats, vitamin E, and antioxidants, which can support brain function.

Dark Chocolate: Dark chocolate contains flavonoids that may enhance memory and cognitive function.

Leafy Greens: Spinach, kale, and other leafy greens are rich in antioxidants and nutrients that support brain health.

Including these brain-boosting foods in the diet can help support cognitive function and brain health.

16.3 Omega-3 Fatty Acids and Brain Health

Omega-3 fatty acids, particularly docosahexaenoic acid (DHA) and eicosapentaenoic acid (EPA), are crucial for brain health. DHA is a major component of brain cell membranes, and EPA has anti-inflammatory properties that can benefit brain function.

Fatty Fish: Salmon, mackerel, sardines, and trout are excellent sources of omega-3 fatty acids.

Flaxseeds and Chia Seeds: These plant-based sources provide alpha-linolenic acid (ALA), a precursor to DHA and EPA.

Walnuts: Walnuts are rich in ALA and other beneficial nutrients for brain health.

Consuming omega-3-rich foods regularly can support cognitive function and may help reduce the risk of cognitive decline.

16.4 The Impact of Sugar and Processed Foods on Mood

While it's essential to focus on brain-boosting foods, it's equally crucial to consider the impact of certain dietary choices on mental well-being. High consumption of sugar and processed foods has been associated with adverse effects on mood and mental health.

Sugar and Mood Swings: Refined sugars can lead to rapid fluctuations in blood sugar levels, causing mood swings and irritability.

Processed Foods and Inflammation: Processed foods high in trans fats and refined carbohydrates may promote inflammation in the body, which can negatively affect brain health.

Limiting the intake of sugary and processed foods and focusing on whole, nutrient-dense foods can support stable mood and mental well-being.

16.5 B-Vitamins and Neurotransmitter Production

B-vitamins play a critical role in the production of neurotransmitters, which are chemical messengers that facilitate communication between nerve cells in the brain. Neurotransmitters, such as serotonin, dopamine, and GABA, are essential for regulating mood, emotions, and cognitive function.

Folate (Vitamin B9): Folate is involved in the synthesis of neurotransmitters like serotonin and dopamine.

Vitamin B6: This vitamin is essential for converting tryptophan into serotonin and for producing other neurotransmitters.

Vitamin B12: B12 plays a role in myelin formation and helps maintain healthy nerve cells.

A deficiency in B-vitamins can negatively impact neurotransmitter production and potentially contribute to mood disorders. Consuming foods rich in B-vitamins, such as leafy greens, legumes, whole grains, and fortified foods, can support mental well-being.

16.6 The Mediterranean Diet and Mental Health

The Mediterranean diet, inspired by the traditional dietary patterns of countries bordering the Mediterranean Sea, has been associated with numerous health benefits, including positive effects on mental well-being.

Emphasis on Whole Foods: The Mediterranean diet focuses on whole, unprocessed foods, including fruits, vegetables, nuts, seeds, whole grains, and legumes.

Healthy Fats: Olive oil, a key component of the diet, is rich in monounsaturated fats, which are beneficial for brain health.

Fish Consumption: Regular consumption of fatty fish provides omega-3 fatty acids, which support cognitive function.

Antioxidants: The diet is abundant in fruits and vegetables, providing essential antioxidants that protect brain cells.

The Mediterranean diet has been linked to reduced risk of depression and better overall mental health, making it a favorable dietary pattern for supporting emotional well-being.

16.7 The Role of Probiotics in Emotional Well-being

As mentioned earlier, the gut microbiota influences the gut-brain axis and can impact mood and emotional well-being through the production of neurotransmitters and other bioactive compounds.

Probiotics: These beneficial bacteria, found in fermented foods and supplements, can help promote a healthy gut microbiota.

Fermented Foods: Foods like yogurt, kefir, sauerkraut, and kimchi are rich sources of probiotics.

Consuming probiotic-rich foods and supplements can positively influence gut health and potentially improve emotional well-being.

16.8 Nutritional Strategies for Stress Management

Stress can significantly impact mental well-being, and nutrition can play a role in supporting stress management.

Adaptogens: Certain herbs, known as adaptogens, can help the body adapt to stress and support a healthy stress response. Examples include ashwagandha and rhodiola.

Complex Carbohydrates: Carbohydrates can temporarily increase serotonin levels, which can have a calming effect. Opt for whole grains and complex carbohydrates instead of refined sugars.

Moderate Caffeine: While caffeine can provide a temporary boost in energy and alertness, excessive caffeine consumption can exacerbate anxiety. Moderation is key.

Balanced Meals: Eating regular, balanced meals can help stabilize blood sugar levels and reduce the risk of stress-induced mood swings.

Incorporating these nutritional strategies into daily life can support stress management and promote emotional well-being.

16.9 Mindful Eating for a Positive Relationship with Food

Mindful eating involves paying attention to the sensory experience of eating and being fully present during meals. This practice can contribute to a positive relationship with food and improve overall well-being.

Slowing Down: Taking time to savor each bite and eating slowly can promote better digestion and allow for better recognition of hunger and fullness cues.

Tuning into Hunger and Fullness: Mindful eating involves being aware of physical hunger and satiety cues, rather than eating out of emotional or external triggers.

Enjoyment and Gratitude: Focusing on the pleasure of eating and expressing gratitude for nourishing foods can enhance the dining experience.

Mindful eating can help foster a healthy relationship with food, reduce stress-related eating, and improve overall well-being.

16.10 Seeking Professional Help for Mental Health and Nutrition

While nutrition plays a crucial role in supporting mental well-being, it is essential to recognize that it is only one aspect of a holistic approach to mental health. For individuals experiencing mental health challenges, seeking professional help from mental health experts, such as therapists, counselors, or psychiatrists, is essential.

Nutritionists and Dietitians: Working with qualified nutrition professionals can provide personalized dietary recommendations tailored to individual needs and health goals.

Interdisciplinary Approach: Mental health and nutrition professionals can collaborate to develop comprehensive treatment plans that address both mental health and nutritional needs.

Conclusion:

Nutrition plays a significant role in promoting mental well-being, cognitive function, and emotional health. By incorporating brain-boosting foods, omega-3 fatty acids, and a balanced diet rich in nutrients, individuals can support their cognitive performance and mood. Additionally, being mindful of the gut-brain connection, the impact of sugar and processed foods on mood, and the role of B-vitamins in neurotransmitter production can contribute to a positive mental state. The Mediterranean diet and probiotics offer beneficial dietary patterns for promoting emotional well-being and supporting gut health. It is essential to recognize the impact of stress on mental health and incorporate nutritional strategies for stress management. Ultimately, seeking professional help from mental health experts and nutritionists can complement dietary changes and provide comprehensive support for mental well-being. By combining nutrition and mental health practices, individuals can take proactive steps towards achieving a balanced and nourishing lifestyle that supports their mental well-being.

Chapter 17: Nutrition for Healthy Skin, Hair, and Nails

The condition of our skin, hair, and nails can reflect our overall health and well-being. Nutrition plays a significant role in maintaining the health and appearance of these external features. This chapter explores the essential nutrients and dietary patterns that contribute to healthy skin, lustrous hair, and strong nails.

17.1 The Link Between Diet and Skin Health

Our skin is the body's largest organ, and its health is influenced by various internal and external factors, including diet. Nutrient-rich foods can provide the necessary building blocks for skin health, while certain dietary choices can contribute to skin issues.

Antioxidant-Rich Foods: Antioxidants help protect the skin from oxidative stress caused by free radicals. Including colorful fruits and vegetables in the diet can provide a wide range of antioxidants.

Omega-3 Fatty Acids: These healthy fats support skin health by reducing inflammation and maintaining the skin's natural moisture barrier. Fatty fish, chia seeds, and walnuts are excellent sources of omega-3s.

Vitamins and Minerals: Nutrients like vitamin A, vitamin C, vitamin E, zinc, and selenium are vital for skin health, supporting collagen production, and promoting skin repair.

Hydration: Adequate water intake is essential for maintaining skin hydration and promoting a healthy complexion.

17.2 Foods Rich in Antioxidants for Skin Protection

Antioxidants play a critical role in protecting the skin from damage caused by free radicals, which can lead to premature aging and other skin issues. Including antioxidant-rich foods in the diet can provide ample protection for the skin.

Berries: Blueberries, strawberries, raspberries, and blackberries are packed with antioxidants, particularly vitamin C and anthocyanins.

Tomatoes: Tomatoes are a rich source of lycopene, a powerful antioxidant that may protect the skin from sun damage.

Dark Leafy Greens: Spinach, kale, and Swiss chard are abundant in vitamins A, C, and E, as well as other antioxidants that support skin health.

Green Tea: Green tea contains catechins, potent antioxidants that may help protect the skin from UV damage.

Nuts and Seeds: Almonds, sunflower seeds, and pumpkin seeds are excellent sources of vitamin E, a skin-protective antioxidant.

Including a variety of antioxidant-rich foods in the diet can help combat oxidative stress and promote radiant, healthy skin.

17.3 Nutrients for Collagen Production

Collagen is a protein that provides structural support for the skin, promoting elasticity and firmness. Nutrients that support collagen production can contribute to skin health and a youthful appearance.

Vitamin C: Vitamin C is essential for collagen synthesis and plays a crucial role in maintaining skin integrity.

Protein: A diet adequate in high-quality protein provides the amino acids necessary for collagen formation.

Silica: Silica is a mineral that supports collagen production and is found in foods like cucumbers, bell peppers, and oats.

Vitamin A: Vitamin A supports skin health and collagen synthesis.

Consuming a balanced diet with these collagen-promoting nutrients can contribute to healthy, supple skin.

17.4 The Role of Water in Skin Hydration

Hydration is crucial for maintaining skin health, as well-hydrated skin appears plump, radiant, and more youthful. Drinking an adequate amount of water throughout the day is essential for maintaining skin hydration.

Water-Rich Foods: Foods like watermelon, cucumber, and oranges have high water content and can contribute to overall hydration.

Herbal Teas: Herbal teas, such as chamomile and peppermint, are hydrating alternatives to plain water.

Water Consumption Tips: Aim to drink at least 8 cups of water daily and increase intake during hot weather or physical activity.

Proper hydration not only supports skin health but also contributes to the overall functioning of the body.

17.5 Vitamin E and Its Benefits for Hair and Nails

Vitamin E is a potent antioxidant that offers numerous benefits for both hair and nails. Including vitamin E-rich foods in the diet can promote healthy hair growth and strengthen nails.

Almonds: Almonds are an excellent source of vitamin E, promoting hair and nail health.

Sunflower Seeds: Sunflower seeds provide vitamin E, along with other nutrients like biotin and zinc, which are beneficial for hair and nails.

Avocado: Avocado is rich in vitamin E and healthy fats that support hair and nail health.

Olive Oil: Using olive oil in cooking or as a salad dressing can provide vitamin E for overall health, including hair and nails.

A diet with sufficient vitamin E can contribute to lustrous hair and strong, healthy nails.

17.6 Foods that Promote a Clear Complexion

A clear complexion is often associated with healthy, radiant skin. Several foods can contribute to a clear complexion by promoting skin health and reducing inflammation.

Probiotic Foods: Fermented foods like yogurt, kefir, and sauerkraut can support gut health, which may positively impact skin clarity.

Turmeric: The anti-inflammatory properties of turmeric may help reduce redness and blemishes on the skin.

Dark Chocolate: Dark chocolate with a high cocoa content contains antioxidants that may promote skin health.

Zinc-Rich Foods: Zinc is an essential mineral for skin health, and foods like pumpkin seeds, chickpeas, and oysters are rich sources.

Green Vegetables: Leafy greens and green vegetables like broccoli and asparagus provide vitamins and minerals that support skin health.

Including these skin-friendly foods in the diet can contribute to a clear and radiant complexion.

17.7 Nutritional Support for Sun Protection

While sunscreen is crucial for protecting the skin from harmful UV rays, certain foods can provide additional support for sun protection.

Tomatoes: Tomatoes are rich in lycopene, which has been associated with some level of sun protection.

Carotenoid-Rich Foods: Carotenoids, found in orange and red fruits and vegetables, may offer some natural sun protection.

Green Tea: Green tea contains polyphenols that may have a protective effect against UV damage.

Consuming a diet rich in these sun-protective nutrients can complement the use of sunscreen and support overall skin health.

17.8 Collagen Supplements and Their Efficacy

Collagen supplements have gained popularity for their potential benefits for skin, hair, and nail health. These supplements typically come in the form of hydrolyzed collagen, which is more easily absorbed by the body.

Supporting Collagen Production: Collagen supplements may provide additional support for collagen synthesis in the body.

Skin Elasticity: Some studies suggest that collagen supplements may improve skin elasticity and moisture retention.

Hair and Nail Health: Collagen supplements may promote hair growth and strengthen nails.

While some studies show promising results, more research is needed to fully understand the efficacy of collagen supplements for skin, hair, and nail health. As with any supplement, it's essential to consult with a healthcare professional before incorporating collagen supplements into one's routine.

17.9 Foods to Avoid for Healthy Skin

While incorporating skin-friendly foods is crucial, it is also essential to be mindful of certain dietary choices that may negatively impact skin health.

High Glycemic Index Foods: Foods with a high glycemic index can cause blood sugar spikes, potentially contributing to acne and skin inflammation.

Processed Foods: Processed foods often contain added sugars, unhealthy fats, and preservatives that may lead to skin issues.

Excessive Alcohol: Heavy alcohol consumption can dehydrate the body and contribute to skin dryness.

Sugary Beverages: Sugar-sweetened

drinks can lead to blood sugar spikes and potentially affect skin health.

Limiting these skin-detrimental foods and focusing on a balanced, nutrient-dense diet can promote healthy skin.

17.10 Creating a Skin-Nourishing Diet Plan

Creating a skin-nourishing diet plan involves incorporating a variety of nutrient-rich foods that support skin health, hair growth, and nail strength.

A Balanced Plate: Aim to include a variety of colorful fruits and vegetables, lean proteins, whole grains, and healthy fats in each meal.

Hydration: Stay well-hydrated by drinking plenty of water and enjoying hydrating beverages.

Limiting Processed Foods: Reduce the intake of processed foods high in added sugars, unhealthy fats, and preservatives.

Supplements: If necessary, consider adding supplements like vitamin E, biotin, or zinc to support hair and nail health.

Consistency: Healthy skin, hair, and nail improvements often result from consistent dietary choices over time.

A skin-nourishing diet plan that prioritizes nutrient-dense foods can contribute to healthy, radiant skin, lustrous hair, and strong nails. Remember that individual needs may vary, and consulting with a registered dietitian or healthcare professional can provide personalized guidance for optimal results.

Chapter 18: Nutrition for Digestive Health

A healthy digestive system is essential for overall well-being as it plays a vital role in breaking down food, absorbing nutrients, and eliminating waste. Proper nutrition is crucial for maintaining digestive health and supporting a balanced gut microbiome. This chapter explores various aspects of nutrition that contribute to optimal digestive function and offers guidelines for building a gut-friendly diet.

18.1 Understanding the Digestive System

The digestive system is a complex network of organs and processes responsible for the breakdown of food and the absorption of nutrients. It includes the mouth, esophagus, stomach, small intestine, large intestine, and anus.

Digestion Process: The process begins in the mouth, where food is chewed and mixed with saliva. It then travels through the esophagus to the stomach, where stomach acids and enzymes help break down the food further. The partially digested food moves to the small intestine, where nutrients are absorbed into the bloodstream. The remaining waste passes to the large intestine for further water absorption and waste elimination.

Factors Affecting Digestion: Digestive health can be influenced by various factors, including diet, hydration, gut microbiota, stress, and physical activity.

18.2 Fiber and Its Role in Digestion

Fiber is a type of carbohydrate found in plant-based foods that the body cannot fully digest. Despite not being absorbed, fiber plays a crucial role in maintaining digestive health.

Promoting Regular Bowel Movements: Insoluble fiber adds bulk to stool, aiding in regular bowel movements and preventing constipation.

Feeding Beneficial Gut Bacteria: Soluble fiber serves as food for beneficial gut bacteria, promoting a healthy gut microbiome.

Supporting Gut Health: Fiber supports overall gut health by preventing inflammation and supporting proper digestion.

Fiber-Rich Foods: Whole grains, fruits, vegetables, legumes, nuts, and seeds are excellent sources of fiber.

18.3 Probiotics and Gut Microbiota

Probiotics are beneficial bacteria that can positively influence the gut microbiota—the diverse community of microorganisms residing in the digestive tract.

Improving Gut Balance: Probiotics can help restore the balance of beneficial bacteria in the gut, which is essential for optimal digestion and immune function.

Supporting Digestive Health: Probiotics have been linked to reduced symptoms of digestive disorders, such as irritable bowel syndrome (IBS) and inflammatory bowel disease (IBD).

Fermented Foods: Yogurt, kefir, sauerkraut, kimchi, and kombucha are examples of fermented foods rich in probiotics.

Probiotic Supplements: Probiotic supplements can be beneficial, especially after a course of antibiotics or for individuals with digestive issues.

18.4 Prebiotics for Gut Health

Prebiotics are non-digestible fibers that serve as food for probiotics, promoting their growth and activity in the gut.

Promoting Beneficial Bacteria: Prebiotics support the growth of beneficial gut bacteria, contributing to a healthy gut microbiome.

Digestive Health: By supporting gut bacteria, prebiotics can improve digestion and nutrient absorption.

Prebiotic-Rich Foods: Onions, garlic, leeks, bananas, asparagus, and chicory root are examples of prebiotic-rich foods.

18.5 The Impact of Fats on Digestive Function

Dietary fats can significantly influence digestive health and function, depending on their type and quantity.

Healthy Fats: Monounsaturated and polyunsaturated fats, found in avocados, olive oil, nuts, and fatty fish, are beneficial for digestive health.

Omega-3 Fatty Acids: Omega-3s have anti-inflammatory properties and may benefit individuals with inflammatory digestive disorders.

Moderation: While healthy fats are beneficial, excessive consumption of unhealthy saturated and trans fats can negatively affect digestion.

18.6 Hydration and Bowel Regularity

Adequate hydration is essential for maintaining bowel regularity and preventing constipation.

Water Absorption: Hydration helps the large intestine absorb water, softening stool and supporting regular bowel movements.

Fluid Balance: Proper hydration helps prevent dehydration, which can lead to digestive discomfort.

Hydrating Foods: Water-rich foods like cucumbers, watermelon, and oranges can contribute to overall hydration.

18.7 Foods for Managing Digestive Disorders

For individuals with specific digestive disorders, certain dietary modifications may be beneficial.

IBS: A low-FODMAP diet, which restricts certain fermentable carbohydrates, may help alleviate IBS symptoms.

IBD: For individuals with inflammatory bowel disease, a diet rich in anti-inflammatory foods and low in trigger foods can be beneficial.

Lactose Intolerance: Limiting lactose-containing foods or using lactase enzyme supplements can help manage lactose intolerance.

Individualized Approach: It's essential for individuals with digestive disorders to work with a registered dietitian to create a personalized diet plan.

18.8 Gluten Sensitivity and Digestive Health

Gluten sensitivity, including celiac disease, is an autoimmune condition triggered by the consumption of gluten, a protein found in wheat, barley, and rye.

Celiac Disease: Individuals with celiac disease must strictly avoid gluten to prevent intestinal damage and associated symptoms.

Non-Celiac Gluten Sensitivity: Some individuals may experience digestive discomfort or other symptoms in response to gluten without having celiac disease.

Gluten-Free Diet: A gluten-free diet involves avoiding all sources of gluten, including wheat, barley, rye, and cross-contaminated products.

18.9 Foods to Soothe an Upset Stomach

Certain foods and remedies can help soothe an upset stomach and alleviate digestive discomfort.

Ginger: Ginger has anti-inflammatory properties and can help alleviate nausea and indigestion.

Peppermint: Peppermint tea or oil may relieve digestive discomfort and bloating.

Bananas and Rice: The BRAT diet, consisting of bananas, rice, applesauce, and toast, can be helpful for easing diarrhea.

Proper Hydration: Staying hydrated with water, herbal teas, or clear broths is essential for managing an upset stomach.

18.10 Building a Gut-Friendly Diet

Creating a gut-friendly diet involves incorporating a variety of nutrient-rich foods that support digestive health and a balanced gut microbiome.

Fiber-Rich Foods: Incorporate a variety of fruits, vegetables, whole grains, and legumes to ensure adequate fiber intake.

Probiotic Foods: Include fermented foods like yogurt, kefir, sauerkraut, and kimchi to support beneficial gut bacteria.

Prebiotic Foods: Onions, garlic, asparagus, and bananas are excellent sources of prebiotic fibers.

Healthy Fats: Incorporate sources of healthy

fats like avocados, nuts, seeds, and fatty fish into the diet.

Hydration: Stay adequately hydrated with water and hydrating foods to support bowel regularity.

Balanced Diet: Aim for a balanced diet that includes a variety of nutrients to support overall digestive health.

By paying attention to the types of foods consumed, the overall dietary pattern, and the inclusion of gut-friendly foods, individuals can promote digestive health and maintain a balanced gut microbiome. As with any dietary change, individual needs may vary, and seeking guidance from a registered dietitian can provide personalized recommendations for optimizing digestive health.

Chapter 19: Nutrition for Bone Health

Bones are the structural framework of the body, providing support, protection, and mobility. Proper nutrition is vital for maintaining strong and healthy bones throughout life. This chapter explores the essential nutrients and dietary factors that contribute to optimal bone health and offers guidelines for preventing osteoporosis and supporting bone healing.

19.1 Understanding Bone Composition and Remodeling

Bones are complex living tissues made up of a matrix of minerals, collagen, and living bone cells. Bone remodeling is a continuous process of breaking down old bone tissue and replacing it with new bone tissue, maintaining bone strength and density.

Osteoblasts and Osteoclasts: Osteoblasts are bone-building cells, while osteoclasts are responsible for bone resorption (breakdown).

Collagen: Collagen provides flexibility and tensile strength to bones, preventing them from becoming too brittle.

Calcium and Phosphorus: Minerals like calcium and phosphorus form the rigid structure of bones, providing strength.

19.2 Calcium and Its Role in Bone Structure

Calcium is a critical mineral for bone health, accounting for about 99% of the body's total calcium content.

Bone Structure: Calcium combines with other minerals to form hydroxyapatite crystals, giving bones their strength and rigidity.

Blood Calcium Levels: If dietary calcium is insufficient, the body may draw calcium from bones to maintain blood calcium levels, weakening bones over time.

Calcium-Rich Foods: Dairy products, leafy greens, almonds, and fortified plant-based milk are good sources of calcium.

19.3 Vitamin D and Bone Health

Vitamin D is essential for bone health as it facilitates calcium absorption and helps maintain proper blood calcium levels.

Calcium Absorption: Vitamin D enhances the absorption of calcium in the intestines, supporting bone mineralization.

Sun Exposure: The skin can synthesize vitamin D when exposed to sunlight, making sun exposure an important factor in bone health.

Food Sources: Fatty fish, fortified dairy products, and egg yolks are dietary sources of vitamin D.

Supplementation: Individuals with limited sun exposure or inadequate dietary intake may benefit from vitamin D supplements.

19.4 Magnesium and Its Impact on Bone Density

Magnesium is a mineral that plays a role in bone metabolism and bone density regulation.

Bone Formation: Magnesium is involved in converting vitamin D into its active form, promoting calcium absorption for bone mineralization.

Bone Density: Studies have shown that higher magnesium intake is associated with increased bone mineral density.

Magnesium-Rich Foods: Nuts, seeds, whole grains, leafy greens, and legumes are excellent sources of magnesium.

19.5 Phosphorus and Other Bone-Building Minerals

Phosphorus is another essential mineral for bone health, accounting for about 80% of the body's total phosphorus content.

Mineral Balance: Calcium and phosphorus work together to maintain bone structure and bone mineralization.

Dietary Sources: Phosphorus is abundant in foods like dairy products, meat, fish, poultry, and nuts.

Other Bone-Building Minerals: Other minerals like potassium, zinc, and copper also play a role in bone health and bone metabolism.

19.6 Protein and Collagen for Bone Strength

Protein is a crucial component of bone tissue, providing the framework for bone structure.

Collagen Matrix: Collagen, the most abundant protein in the body, provides flexibility and strength to bones.

Bone Density: Low protein intake can negatively affect bone density and bone health.

Sources of Protein: Lean meats, poultry, fish, legumes, nuts, and dairy products are excellent sources of protein.

19.7 Vitamin K and Bone Health

Vitamin K is essential for bone health as it activates proteins involved in bone mineralization.

Calcium Regulation: Vitamin K supports calcium utilization in bone tissue, contributing to bone strength.

Bone Health Benefits: Studies suggest that vitamin K intake is associated with improved bone health and reduced fracture risk.

Vitamin K-Rich Foods: Leafy greens, broccoli, Brussels sprouts, and fermented foods are good sources of vitamin K.

19.8 Foods for Osteoporosis Prevention

Osteoporosis is a bone disease characterized by low bone mass and increased bone fragility. Proper nutrition plays a crucial role in preventing osteoporosis.

Calcium and Vitamin D: Adequate intake of calcium and vitamin D throughout life is essential for building and maintaining strong bones.

Magnesium: Consuming foods rich in magnesium can support bone density and bone health.

Protein: Ensuring sufficient protein intake can promote bone strength and prevent bone loss.

Vitamin K: Including vitamin K-rich foods can help support bone mineralization and reduce the risk of fractures.

Phytonutrients: Plant-based foods contain phytonutrients that may benefit bone health.

Maintaining a balanced diet rich in nutrients and focusing on bone-building foods can reduce the risk of osteoporosis.

19.9 The Impact of Exercise on Bone Density

Regular weight-bearing and resistance exercises can promote bone health by stimulating bone formation and increasing bone density.

Weight-Bearing Exercises: Activities like walking, jogging, dancing, and hiking put stress on bones, stimulating bone remodeling.

Resistance Training: Strength training exercises, like lifting weights, promote bone density and muscle strength.

Balance and Flexibility: Exercises that improve balance and flexibility can reduce the risk of falls and fractures.

Regular physical activity throughout life can help build and maintain strong bones.

19.10 Nutritional Considerations for Bone Healing

Proper nutrition is essential for bone healing after fractures or injuries.

Calcium and Vitamin D: Adequate intake of calcium and vitamin D supports bone healing and recovery.

Protein: Sufficient protein intake provides the building blocks necessary for bone repair.

Micronutrients: Nutrients like vitamins C, A, and zinc are crucial for collagen synthesis and tissue repair.

Hydration: Staying well-hydrated supports overall healing processes.

During the healing process, focusing on a nutrient-rich diet can aid in bone recovery and support optimal healing.

Conclusion:

Nutrition plays a fundamental role in supporting bone health throughout life. Adequate intake of calcium, vitamin D, magnesium, phosphorus, and other bone-building minerals provides the essential elements for strong bones. Protein and collagen support bone structure and healing

, while vitamin K activates proteins involved in bone mineralization. Including bone-healthy foods, exercising regularly, and maintaining a balanced diet are essential strategies for maintaining optimal bone health and preventing conditions like osteoporosis. As individual needs may vary, consulting with a healthcare professional or registered dietitian can provide personalized guidance for optimizing bone health.

Chapter 20: Nutrition for Weight Management

Weight management is a complex process influenced by various factors, including dietary choices, physical activity, sleep, stress, and emotional well-being. This chapter explores the key elements of nutrition that play a significant role in weight management. From understanding energy balance to adopting mindful eating practices, these guidelines aim to help individuals create a sustainable and healthy approach to weight loss and maintenance.

20.1 Understanding the Factors Influencing Weight

Weight is influenced by a combination of genetic, environmental, and lifestyle factors.

Genetics: Genetic makeup can impact metabolism, fat storage, and hunger cues.

Environment: Access to food, cultural influences, and societal norms play a role in food choices and portion sizes.

Lifestyle: Physical activity levels, sleep patterns, and stress management can affect weight.

20.2 Energy Balance: Calories In vs. Calories Out

Weight management revolves around energy balance, where calories consumed should match the calories expended.

Calories In: This refers to the energy derived from food and beverages consumed.

Calories Out: This includes the energy expended through physical activity, resting metabolic rate, and the thermic effect of food.

Weight Loss: To lose weight, the calories burned should exceed the calories consumed.

Weight Maintenance: To maintain weight, the calories in and out should be balanced.

20.3 The Role of Macronutrients in Weight Loss and Gain

Macronutrients, which include carbohydrates, proteins, and fats, impact energy balance and body composition.

Carbohydrates: High-carb diets may lead to increased insulin levels, potentially promoting fat storage.

Proteins: Protein promotes satiety and helps preserve muscle mass during weight loss.

Fats: Healthy fats support hormone production and fat-soluble vitamin absorption.

Balanced Macronutrient Intake: A balanced diet that includes all three macronutrients in appropriate proportions is essential for weight management.

20.4 Fiber and Satiety: Feeling Full with Fewer Calories

Fiber is a type of carbohydrate that is not fully digested, contributing to feelings of fullness and satiety.

Increased Satiety: High-fiber foods keep individuals feeling full for longer, reducing overall calorie intake.

Regulating Blood Sugar: Fiber helps stabilize blood sugar levels, preventing rapid spikes and crashes in energy.

Fiber-Rich Foods: Fruits, vegetables, whole grains, legumes, and nuts are excellent sources of fiber.

20.5 Protein for Appetite Control and Muscle Preservation

Protein plays a crucial role in weight management, as it supports appetite control and muscle preservation.

Satiety: Protein-rich foods trigger the release of satiety hormones, reducing feelings of hunger.

Muscle Preservation: During weight loss, adequate protein intake helps preserve lean muscle mass.

Sources of Protein: Lean meats, poultry, fish, dairy products, legumes, and plant-based proteins are good sources of protein.

20.6 Managing Emotional Eating and Food Cravings

Emotional eating and food cravings can lead to overeating and weight gain.

Identifying Triggers: Becoming aware of emotional triggers for eating can help individuals develop healthier coping strategies.

Mindfulness Techniques: Practicing mindfulness can help individuals differentiate between physical hunger and emotional eating.

Healthy Coping Mechanisms: Engaging in non-food-related activities to manage emotions, like exercise or hobbies, can be beneficial.

20.7 Balanced Meal Planning for Weight Maintenance

Balanced meal planning involves incorporating a variety of nutrient-dense foods into daily meals.

Portion Control: Controlling portion sizes can prevent overeating and support weight management.

Nutrient-Rich Foods: Prioritize fruits, vegetables, lean proteins, whole grains, and healthy fats in meals.

Regular Eating Patterns: Consistency in meal timing can help regulate hunger cues and prevent overeating.

20.8 Mindful Eating and Portion Control

Mindful eating involves being fully present and aware of the eating experience.

Slowing Down: Eating slowly and savoring each bite can help individuals recognize feelings of fullness.

Portion Awareness: Using smaller plates and bowls can aid in portion control.

Eliminating Distractions: Avoiding distractions like screens while eating can help individuals focus on their meal.

20.9 The Impact of Sleep and Stress on Weight

Both sleep quality and stress levels can affect weight management.

Sleep: Lack of sleep can disrupt hunger hormones, leading to increased appetite and weight gain.

Stress: Chronic stress can trigger emotional eating and promote weight gain.

Prioritizing Sleep: Aim for 7-9 hours of quality sleep per night to support weight management.

Stress Management: Engaging in stress-reducing activities like meditation, yoga, or exercise can be beneficial.

20.10 Creating a Sustainable and Healthy Weight Loss Plan

A successful and sustainable weight loss plan involves setting realistic goals and making gradual changes.

Small Steps: Start with small changes in diet and physical activity to build healthy habits over time.

Realistic Goals: Set achievable weight loss goals based on individual needs and preferences.

Behavior Change: Focus on behavior changes rather than quick-fix diets for long-term success.

Seeking Support: Consulting with a registered dietitian or healthcare professional can provide personalized guidance.

Conclusion:

Weight management is a multifaceted journey that involves understanding energy balance, making informed food choices, practicing mindful eating, and addressing emotional factors. By focusing on balanced nutrition, regular physical activity, adequate sleep, and stress management, individuals can create a sustainable and healthy approach to weight loss and maintenance. Setting realistic goals and seeking professional support when needed can contribute to successful long-term weight management and overall well-being.

Chapter 21: The Role of Mindfulness in Weight Management

21.1 Understanding Mindful Eating

Mindful eating is a practice that involves being fully present and aware of the eating experience. It focuses on paying attention to the taste, texture, and sensations of food, as well as recognizing hunger and fullness cues. Mindful eating encourages individuals to cultivate a non-judgmental attitude towards food and eating habits, leading to a healthier relationship with food.

The Benefits of Mindful Eating: Mindful eating can help individuals become more attuned to their body's signals, prevent overeating, and improve overall satisfaction with meals.

21.2 Mindfulness Techniques for Curbing Emotional Eating

Emotional eating is the tendency to use food to cope with emotions rather than eating in response to physical hunger. Mindfulness techniques can be powerful tools for curbing emotional eating.

Recognizing Emotional Triggers: Mindfulness helps individuals become aware of emotional triggers that lead to overeating.

Finding Alternative Coping Strategies: Practicing mindfulness can help individuals identify healthier ways to cope with emotions, such as deep breathing, meditation, or engaging in enjoyable activities.

21.3 The Connection Between Mindfulness and Satiety

Mindful eating can enhance the sense of satiety during and after meals. By being fully present while eating, individuals can better recognize feelings of fullness and satisfaction.

Eating Slower: Eating slowly allows the brain to register feelings of fullness, preventing overeating.

Listening to Hunger Cues: Mindful eating helps individuals tune into their body's hunger and fullness signals.

Choosing Nutrient-Dense Foods: Being mindful of food choices can lead to selecting nutrient-dense options that provide greater satisfaction.

21.4 Mindful Meal Planning and Preparation

Meal planning and preparation can be mindful practices that foster a positive and enjoyable relationship with food.

Planning Balanced Meals: Mindful meal planning involves incorporating a variety of nutrient-rich foods into each meal.

Savoring the Cooking Process: Taking pleasure in the process of cooking can increase appreciation for the food being prepared.

21.5 Mindfulness-Based Stress Reduction for Weight Loss

Stress can contribute to weight gain and hinder weight loss efforts. Mindfulness-based stress reduction (MBSR) techniques can help manage stress and improve overall well-being.

Meditation: Regular meditation can reduce stress and emotional eating tendencies.

Yoga: Practicing yoga can help lower stress levels and increase mindfulness.

21.6 The Impact of Mindfulness on Food Choices

Mindful eating can influence food choices by encouraging individuals to make more conscious and healthful decisions.

Increased Awareness: Mindfulness heightens awareness of the impact of food choices on well-being.

Reduced Impulse Eating: Being mindful can help individuals resist impulsive and unhealthy food choices.

21.7 Practicing Mindful Eating in Social Settings

Mindful eating can be practiced in social settings and during special occasions.

Staying Present: Being mindful of the eating experience in social settings can prevent mindless overeating.

Balancing Indulgences: Mindful eating allows individuals to enjoy treats in moderation without guilt.

21.8 Mindful Exercise: Finding Joy in Physical Activity

Mindfulness can be applied to exercise routines to enhance enjoyment and promote regular physical activity.

Tuning into the Body: Being mindful during exercise helps individuals tune into their body's signals and avoid pushing past their limits.

Discovering Enjoyable Activities: Engaging in physical activities that bring joy can increase motivation to stay active.

21.9 Overcoming Plateaus with Mindfulness

Weight loss plateaus can be frustrating, but mindfulness can help individuals navigate through these challenges.

Practicing Patience: Mindfulness fosters patience and self-compassion during weight loss plateaus.

Reflecting on Progress: Being mindful of progress beyond the number on the scale can boost motivation.

21.10 Creating a Mindfulness Routine for Sustainable Weight Loss

Incorporating mindfulness into daily routines can support long-term and sustainable weight loss.

Mindful Eating Habits: Practicing mindful eating at every meal helps create a healthy relationship with food.

Mindful Movement: Incorporating mindfulness into physical activities promotes regular exercise and reduces stress.

Conclusion:

Mindfulness is a powerful practice that can positively impact weight management. By being fully present and aware of the eating experience, individuals can develop healthier eating habits, recognize emotional triggers for overeating, and better understand their body's hunger and fullness cues. Mindfulness can also reduce stress, enhance enjoyment in physical activities, and provide tools for navigating weight loss plateaus. Incorporating mindfulness into daily routines creates a sustainable and mindful approach to weight management, promoting overall well-being and a positive relationship with food and body.

Chapter 22: Nutrition for Hormonal Balance and Weight

Hormonal balance plays a crucial role in weight management, influencing appetite, metabolism, and body composition. This chapter explores the impact of various hormones on weight and offers nutrition strategies to support hormonal balance for sustainable weight management.

22.1 Understanding Hormones and Their Impact on Weight

Hormones are chemical messengers produced by various glands in the body, regulating essential functions, including metabolism, hunger, and fat storage.

Leptin and Ghrelin: These hormones control hunger and satiety signals, affecting appetite and food intake.

Insulin: Insulin regulates blood sugar levels and influences fat storage.

Estrogen, Progesterone, and Testosterone: These sex hormones impact fat distribution and metabolism.

Cortisol: The stress hormone cortisol can lead to increased appetite and fat storage.

Thyroid Hormones: Thyroid hormones control metabolism and energy expenditure.

Hormonal imbalances can lead to weight gain or hinder weight loss efforts.

22.2 The Role of Insulin in Weight Management

Insulin is a hormone produced by the pancreas that regulates blood sugar levels and fat storage.

Insulin Resistance: In insulin resistance, cells become less responsive to insulin, leading to higher blood sugar levels and increased fat storage.

Fat Storage: Excess insulin can promote fat storage, particularly around the abdominal area.

Balancing Insulin: Consuming balanced meals with a mix of carbohydrates, proteins, and healthy fats can help stabilize blood sugar levels.

22.3 Balancing Estrogen and Weight

Estrogen is a hormone primarily associated with female reproductive health, but it also influences weight.

Estrogen Dominance: High levels of estrogen relative to other hormones can contribute to weight gain.

Metabolism: Estrogen plays a role in metabolic rate and fat distribution.

Estrogen Balance: Consuming phytoestrogen-rich foods, like flaxseeds and soy products, can help balance estrogen levels.

22.4 Progesterone and Its Influence on Appetite

Progesterone, another female sex hormone, can influence appetite and weight.

Appetite Regulation: Progesterone may have a mild appetite-suppressing effect.

Fluid Retention: Progesterone can cause water retention, leading to temporary weight gain.

Natural Strategies: Maintaining a balanced diet and managing stress can support progesterone balance.

22.5 Testosterone and Its Effect on Body Composition

Testosterone is the primary male sex hormone, but it also plays a role in female health.

Muscle Mass: Testosterone supports muscle growth and preservation, influencing body composition.

Fat Loss: Adequate testosterone levels can aid in fat loss and weight management.

Resistance Training: Engaging in resistance training can naturally boost testosterone levels.

22.6 Cortisol, Stress, and Weight Gain

Cortisol, the stress hormone, can impact appetite, food choices, and fat storage.

Stress Eating: High cortisol levels can lead to emotional eating and cravings for unhealthy foods.

Visceral Fat: Chronic stress is associated with increased visceral fat, which surrounds internal organs and poses health risks.

Stress Management: Mindfulness techniques, exercise, and relaxation practices can help manage stress and cortisol levels.

22.7 The Thyroid-Weight Connection

Thyroid hormones, particularly T3 and T4, regulate metabolism and energy expenditure.

Hypothyroidism: An underactive thyroid can lead to weight gain and difficulty losing weight.

Hyperthyroidism: An overactive thyroid can lead to weight loss and difficulty gaining weight.

Balancing Thyroid Function: Consuming sufficient iodine, selenium, and other nutrients is essential for thyroid health.

22.8 Foods that Support Hormonal Balance

A balanced diet rich in nutrients can support hormonal balance and weight management.

Phytonutrients: Plant-based foods, such as fruits, vegetables, and whole grains, contain phytonutrients that support hormone metabolism.

Healthy Fats: Omega-3 fatty acids and monounsaturated fats can support hormonal health.

Fiber: A high-fiber diet can help regulate blood sugar levels and support hormonal balance.

22.9 Exercise and Hormonal Regulation

Regular physical activity can positively impact hormone levels and weight management.

Resistance Training: Strength training can increase testosterone and support muscle growth.

Aerobic Exercise: Cardiovascular exercise can improve insulin sensitivity and support fat loss.

Stress Reduction: Exercise can reduce stress and cortisol levels.

22.10 Seeking Professional Guidance for Hormonal Imbalances

If individuals suspect hormonal imbalances affecting weight, it is essential to consult healthcare professionals.

Hormone Testing: Blood tests can identify hormonal imbalances and guide treatment.

Registered Dietitians and Nutritionists: These professionals can offer personalized dietary strategies to support hormonal balance.

Hormone Replacement Therapy: In some cases, hormone replacement therapy may be necessary to address imbalances.

Conclusion:

Hormonal balance is a critical factor in weight management, influencing appetite, metabolism, and body composition. Understanding the impact of hormones on weight and adopting appropriate nutrition and lifestyle strategies can support hormonal health and sustainable weight management. By embracing balanced meals, managing stress, engaging in regular exercise, and seeking professional guidance when necessary,

individuals can optimize hormonal function and achieve their weight management goals.

Chapter 23: Intermittent Fasting and Weight Loss

Intermittent fasting has gained popularity as a weight loss approach in recent years. This chapter explores the concept of intermittent fasting, its various types, benefits for weight loss, effects on metabolism and insulin sensitivity, as well as potential risks and considerations. Additionally, it provides guidance on combining intermittent fasting with balanced nutrition and designing a suitable fasting schedule.

23.1 Understanding Intermittent Fasting

Intermittent fasting is an eating pattern that alternates between periods of eating and fasting.

Fasting Periods: During fasting, individuals abstain from calorie intake, giving the body a chance to rest and reset.

Feeding Windows: Intermittent fasting is structured around feeding windows, limiting the time when meals are consumed.

23.2 The Different Types of Intermittent Fasting

There are several intermittent fasting methods, each with its own fasting and feeding durations.

16/8 Method: Involves fasting for 16 hours and eating during an 8-hour window each day.

5:2 Method: Involves eating normally for five days and significantly reducing calorie intake (about 500-600 calories) on two non-consecutive days.

Alternate-Day Fasting: Involves alternating between fasting days and regular eating days.

Eat-Stop-Eat: Involves fasting for 24 hours once or twice a week.

Warrior Diet: Involves fasting during the day and eating a large meal at night.

23.3 The Benefits of Intermittent Fasting for Weight Loss

Intermittent fasting offers several potential benefits for weight loss.

Caloric Restriction: Intermittent fasting naturally limits calorie intake, promoting a caloric deficit.

Fat Burning: During fasting periods, the body may use stored fat as an energy source.

Improved Hormonal Balance: Intermittent fasting can influence hormones related to hunger and metabolism.

23.4 Intermittent Fasting and Its Impact on Metabolism

Intermittent fasting may affect metabolic processes in the body.

Autophagy: Fasting induces autophagy, a process that helps remove damaged cells and may promote longevity.

Insulin Sensitivity: Intermittent fasting can improve insulin sensitivity, which is beneficial for weight management.

Resting Metabolic Rate: Some studies suggest that intermittent fasting may not negatively impact resting metabolic rate.

23.5 Combining Intermittent Fasting with Balanced Nutrition

To reap the full benefits of intermittent fasting, it is essential to combine it with balanced and nutritious eating habits.

Nutrient-Dense Foods: Focus on consuming whole, nutrient-dense foods during feeding windows.

Avoid Overeating: Even during feeding windows, avoid excessive calorie intake that might negate fasting benefits.

Stay Hydrated: Drink plenty of water during fasting periods to stay hydrated.

23.6 Managing Hunger and Cravings during Fasting Periods

Hunger and cravings may arise during fasting periods, and several strategies can help manage them.

Stay Hydrated: Drinking water, herbal teas, or black coffee can help curb hunger.

Mindful Eating: Be present and mindful during feeding windows to fully enjoy meals and prevent overeating.

Include Satiating Foods: Incorporate protein, healthy fats, and fiber-rich foods to promote satiety.

23.7 Intermittent Fasting for Improving Insulin Sensitivity

Intermittent fasting can positively impact insulin sensitivity, a crucial factor in weight management and overall health.

Balanced Blood Sugar: Intermittent fasting may help stabilize blood sugar levels.

Reduced Insulin Resistance: Fasting periods can reduce insulin resistance, improving the body's response to insulin.

23.8 Potential Risks and Considerations of Intermittent Fasting

Intermittent fasting may not be suitable for everyone, and some individuals should approach it with caution.

Individual Differences: Intermittent fasting may have different effects on various individuals.

Medical Conditions: People with certain medical conditions should consult a healthcare professional before attempting intermittent fasting.

Disordered Eating: Intermittent fasting may not be appropriate for individuals with a history of disordered eating.

23.9 Designing an Intermittent Fasting Schedule

Designing a personalized intermittent fasting schedule requires consideration of lifestyle, daily routines, and individual preferences.

Ease into Fasting: Gradually increase fasting periods to allow the body to adjust.

Find a Feeding Window: Determine the feeding window that fits your lifestyle and preferences.

Experiment and Adapt: Be open to adjusting the fasting schedule based on how your body responds.

23.10 Listening to Your Body: Finding the Right Approach for You

As with any dietary approach, it is crucial to listen to your body's signals and adjust accordingly.

Be Flexible: Be flexible with intermittent fasting, adapting it to fit your needs and goals.

Consider Lifestyle: Choose an intermittent fasting approach that aligns with your lifestyle and daily routines.

Conclusion:

Intermittent fasting can be an effective tool for weight management, but it may not be suitable for everyone. Understanding the different types of intermittent fasting, the potential benefits, and considerations will help individuals make informed decisions about incorporating intermittent fasting into their lifestyle. Combining intermittent fasting with balanced nutrition and listening to your body's signals can contribute to successful weight loss and overall well-being

. Before starting any fasting regimen, it is advisable to consult with a healthcare professional, especially if you have any underlying health conditions or concerns.

Chapter 24: Nutrition for Emotional Well-Being and Weight

Emotional eating can significantly impact weight management, leading to weight gain or hindered weight loss efforts. This chapter explores the connection between emotions and eating habits, strategies for identifying emotional eating triggers, and the role of mindful eating in providing emotional support. Additionally, it delves into the impact of comfort foods on mood, the importance of developing healthy coping mechanisms, seeking support for emotional eating challenges, and nourishing the mind-body connection for better mental health.

24.1 Emotional Eating and Weight Gain

Emotional eating refers to the consumption of food in response to emotions rather than physical hunger.

Comfort Eating: Emotional eaters often turn to comfort foods to cope with stress, sadness, or other emotional challenges.

Weight Gain: Frequent emotional eating can lead to weight gain and difficulties in managing weight.

24.2 Identifying Triggers for Emotional Eating

Identifying emotional eating triggers is crucial in breaking the cycle of emotional eating.

Stress and Anxiety: Stress and anxiety can trigger emotional eating as a way to seek comfort or distraction.

Loneliness and Boredom: Feelings of loneliness or boredom may lead to mindless snacking or overeating.

Negative Emotions: Emotional eaters may turn to food to cope with sadness, anger, or frustration.

24.3 Mindful Eating for Emotional Support

Mindful eating practices can provide emotional support and prevent emotional eating.

Pause and Assess: Before eating, pause and assess if you are physically hungry or responding to emotions.

Eat Without Distractions: Avoid eating while watching TV or using electronic devices to stay mindful.

Savor Each Bite: Take time to savor the flavors and textures of the food to enhance the eating experience.

24.4 The Impact of Comfort Foods on Mood

Comfort foods, often high in sugar and fat, can temporarily improve mood due to the release of "feel-good" neurotransmitters.

Serotonin Boost: Certain comfort foods can increase serotonin levels, promoting a sense of well-being.

Dopamine Release: Foods high in sugar and fat can trigger the release of dopamine, creating a pleasurable sensation.

24.5 Developing Healthy Coping Mechanisms

Finding alternative coping mechanisms to deal with emotions can help break the cycle of emotional eating.

Physical Activity: Engaging in physical activities can reduce stress and boost mood.

Mindfulness Practices: Meditation, yoga, or deep breathing exercises can help manage emotions.

Creative Outlets: Pursuing creative hobbies can serve as a healthy emotional outlet.

24.6 Emotional Awareness and Its Effect on Eating Habits

Becoming more emotionally aware can help individuals recognize patterns of emotional eating.

Keeping a Food Journal: Maintaining a food journal can help identify emotional triggers related to eating.

Emotional Self-Reflection: Regularly reflecting on emotions and eating habits can foster emotional awareness.

24.7 Seeking Support for Emotional Eating Challenges

Seeking support from friends, family, or professionals can be beneficial in managing emotional eating challenges.

Talk to Loved Ones: Share your struggles with loved ones to gain understanding and encouragement.

Professional Guidance: Seek the support of a therapist, counselor, or registered dietitian for personalized assistance.

24.8 Nourishing the Mind-Body Connection

Nourishing the mind-body connection is essential for overall well-being and weight management.

Regular Exercise: Physical activity not only supports weight management but also improves mental health.

Adequate Sleep: Getting enough sleep is crucial for emotional regulation and weight management.

Mindfulness and Meditation: Incorporating mindfulness and meditation practices can reduce emotional eating tendencies.

24.9 Nutrition and Mental Health

Nutrition plays a significant role in supporting mental health and emotional well-being.

Balanced Diet: A balanced diet with essential nutrients can promote emotional stability.

Omega-3 Fatty Acids: Omega-3s are linked to improved mood and reduced risk of depression.

Probiotics: Gut health and mental health are connected, and probiotics can positively influence mood.

24.10 Creating a Positive Relationship with Food and Self

Developing a positive relationship with food and self-esteem is vital for long-term emotional well-being and weight management.

Practice Self-Compassion: Be kind to yourself and avoid self-criticism related to eating habits.

Cultivate Positive Eating Habits: Focus on nourishing the body with healthy foods and enjoying meals mindfully.

Address Emotional Needs: Seek emotional support and develop healthy coping mechanisms for emotional challenges.

Conclusion:

Emotional eating can significantly impact weight management, but by identifying triggers, practicing mindful eating, and developing healthy coping mechanisms, individuals can break the cycle of emotional eating. Additionally, nourishing the mind-body connection, seeking support when needed, and cultivating a positive relationship with food and self can support emotional well-being and lead to a healthier approach to eating and weight management. Combining nutritional strategies with emotional awareness can create a holistic approach to overall well-being.

Chapter 25: Nutrition for a Healthy Gut Microbiome and Weight

The gut microbiome plays a crucial role in various aspects of health, including weight regulation. This chapter explores the significance of the gut microbiome, its influence on weight management, and the impact of prebiotics, probiotics, and fermented foods on gut health. Additionally, it delves into the gut-brain axis and its connection to appetite, foods that promote beneficial gut bacteria, and the link between gut health and inflammation. Furthermore, it discusses the potential role of probiotics in weight management, addressing gut dysbiosis for improved weight control, and cultivating a gut-friendly diet to support weight loss efforts.

25.1 The Gut Microbiome and Its Importance

The gut microbiome consists of trillions of microorganisms residing in the digestive tract.

Microbial Diversity: A diverse gut microbiome is vital for overall health and well-being.

Digestion and Absorption: Gut bacteria aid in the digestion and absorption of nutrients.

Immune Function: The gut microbiome plays a critical role in supporting the immune system.

25.2 How Gut Bacteria Affect Weight Regulation

The gut microbiome can influence weight regulation through various mechanisms.

Energy Harvesting: Certain gut bacteria can extract more calories from food, potentially contributing to weight gain.

Metabolism Regulation: The gut microbiome may impact metabolism and fat storage.

Inflammation: An imbalanced microbiome can lead to chronic low-grade inflammation, which may affect weight.

25.3 Prebiotics and Probiotics for Gut Health

Prebiotics and probiotics are essential for nurturing a healthy gut microbiome.

Prebiotics: Prebiotics are non-digestible fibers that promote the growth of beneficial gut bacteria.

Probiotics: Probiotics are live beneficial bacteria that can be consumed through food or supplements.

25.4 Fermented Foods and Their Impact on the Microbiome

Fermented foods are rich in probiotics and can positively influence the gut microbiome.

Yogurt: Yogurt contains live cultures that contribute to a healthy gut.

Kimchi: Kimchi is a traditional Korean fermented vegetable dish with probiotic properties.

Kefir: Kefir is a fermented milk drink rich in probiotics.

25.5 The Gut-Brain Axis and Its Influence on Appetite

The gut-brain axis refers to the bidirectional communication between the gut and the brain.

Appetite Regulation: Gut bacteria can influence hormones that regulate appetite.

Mood and Behavior: The gut microbiome can impact mood and behavior, which may influence eating habits.

25.6 Foods that Nourish Beneficial Gut Bacteria

Certain foods can nourish and support the growth of beneficial gut bacteria.

High-Fiber Foods: Whole grains, fruits, and vegetables are excellent sources of prebiotic fibers.

Polyphenol-Rich Foods: Polyphenols in foods like berries and dark chocolate can promote gut health.

25.7 The Connection Between Gut Health and Inflammation

An imbalanced gut microbiome can lead to chronic inflammation, which may contribute to weight gain.

Inflammation and Weight: Chronic inflammation can disrupt metabolic processes and contribute to weight gain.

Anti-Inflammatory Foods: Foods rich in omega-3 fatty acids and antioxidants can help reduce inflammation.

25.8 Probiotics and Their Potential Role in Weight Management

Probiotics may have a role in supporting weight management.

Weight Loss: Some studies suggest that certain probiotics may aid in weight loss.

Metabolic Health: Probiotics may improve insulin sensitivity and lipid profiles.

25.9 Addressing Gut Dysbiosis for Improved Weight Control

Gut dysbiosis refers to an imbalance in the gut microbiome, which can affect weight control.

Dietary Interventions: Adopting a balanced and diverse diet can promote a healthy gut microbiome.

Reducing Sugar and Processed Foods: High sugar and processed foods can disrupt gut bacteria and should be limited.

25.10 Cultivating a Gut-Friendly Diet for Weight Loss

A gut-friendly diet can support weight loss efforts and overall well-being.

Balanced Diet: Focus on a balanced diet with a variety of nutrient-dense foods.

Probiotic-Rich Foods: Incorporate probiotic-rich foods like yogurt and fermented vegetables into your diet.

Prebiotic Foods: Include prebiotic-rich foods like oats, bananas, and garlic to support beneficial gut bacteria.

Conclusion:

A healthy gut microbiome is essential for overall health and can significantly impact weight regulation. Including probiotic-rich foods, prebiotic fibers, and fermented foods in the diet can support gut health. The gut-brain axis also plays a role in appetite regulation, making mindfulness and stress management important for weight management. Reducing inflammation through a nutrient-dense diet can further support weight loss efforts. By understanding the significance of the gut microbiome and adopting a gut-friendly diet, individuals can take proactive steps towards improving gut health and achieving their weight management goals. As always, personalized guidance from healthcare professionals or registered dietitians can aid in developing an individualized plan for optimal gut health and weight control.

Chapter 26: Nutritional Strategies for Breaking Through Plateaus

Chapter 26: Nutritional Strategies for Breaking Through Plateaus

Weight loss plateaus are common and can be frustrating for many individuals on a weight loss journey. After making significant progress, it's not uncommon to hit a point where the scale stops budging. However, understanding why plateaus occur and implementing the right nutritional strategies can help break through these obstacles and continue making progress towards your weight loss goals. In this chapter, we will explore various approaches to overcome weight loss plateaus and stay motivated on your weight loss journey.

26.1 Understanding Weight Loss Plateaus

A weight loss plateau refers to a period during a weight loss journey when the rate of weight loss slows down significantly or even stops altogether. It often occurs after experiencing initial success, leaving many individuals feeling discouraged and unsure about how to proceed. Plateaus can be caused by various factors, including metabolic adaptations, changes in body composition, and the body's natural defense mechanisms against perceived starvation.

26.2 The Science behind Plateauing Weight

Several physiological and psychological factors contribute to weight loss plateaus. One primary factor is metabolic adaptation, where the body adjusts its metabolism in response to reduced calorie intake and weight loss. As you lose weight, your body requires fewer calories to function, leading to a decline in the rate of weight loss. Additionally, the body tends to preserve energy by reducing non-essential functions, which can further slow down weight loss.

Changes in body composition can also affect weight loss progress. As you lose weight, you may experience a decrease in muscle mass, which can lead to a decline in resting metabolic rate. Since muscles require more energy to maintain than fat, a reduction in muscle mass can contribute to a slowdown in weight loss.

Moreover, psychological factors, such as stress and emotional eating, can play a role in weight loss plateaus. Stress can lead to hormonal imbalances that may influence appetite and fat storage. Emotional eating can also derail progress by causing individuals to consume excess calories, hindering weight loss efforts.

26.3 Reassessing Your Caloric Needs and Intake

When faced with a weight loss plateau, it's crucial to reassess your caloric needs and intake. As your body weight changes, your caloric requirements may also shift. Recalculate your Total Daily Energy Expenditure (TDEE) based on your current weight, activity level, and goals. Adjusting your calorie intake to match your new TDEE can help reignite weight loss.

However, be cautious not to slash calories too drastically, as this can lead to nutrient deficiencies and a slowdown in metabolism. Gradual and moderate adjustments to your caloric intake are recommended to ensure sustainable and healthy weight loss.

26.4 Adjusting Macronutrient Ratios for Progress

While total calorie intake is essential, the distribution of macronutrients (carbohydrates, proteins, and fats) can also impact weight loss progress. Consider adjusting the ratio of macronutrients in your diet to see if it helps break through the plateau.

Increasing protein intake can be particularly beneficial, as protein helps preserve muscle mass and boosts satiety, making it easier to control hunger and avoid overeating. Including more lean sources of protein like poultry, fish, legumes, and tofu can support your weight loss efforts.

On the other hand, reducing carbohydrate intake, especially refined sugars and processed foods, may help some individuals overcome plateaus. Low-carb or ketogenic diets have gained popularity for their potential to promote weight loss and fat burning.

However, it's essential to remember that each individual is unique, and there is no one-size-fits-all approach to macronutrient ratios.

Experimenting with different combinations of carbohydrates, proteins, and fats can help you find the right balance that works for your body and helps you break through the plateau.

26.5 Incorporating High-Intensity Interval Training (HIIT)

Exercise is a crucial component of any weight loss plan, and incorporating High-Intensity Interval Training (HIIT) can be especially effective for breaking through plateaus. HIIT involves alternating short bursts of intense exercise with periods of rest or low-intensity activity.

HIIT workouts are time-efficient and can boost metabolism, helping the body burn more calories both during and after the exercise session. This can be particularly helpful when faced with a weight loss plateau, as it revs up the body's energy expenditure and encourages fat burning.

Additionally, HIIT can help preserve muscle mass while promoting fat loss, preventing a decline in resting metabolic rate and enhancing overall weight loss progress.

26.6 Exploring Different Exercise Modalities for Variety

Variety in your exercise routine can be beneficial not only for breaking through plateaus but also for maintaining long-term motivation. Trying out different exercise modalities can challenge your body in new ways, preventing it from adapting to a specific routine.

Consider incorporating strength training, cardio exercises, yoga, Pilates, or other forms of physical activity into your weekly schedule. Cross-training can engage different muscle groups and help you avoid hitting a plateau.

Moreover, engaging in activities you enjoy can make exercise more enjoyable and sustainable. Whether it's dancing, swimming, hiking, or playing a sport, finding activities that bring you joy can help you stay motivated and committed to your weight loss journey.

26.7 Tracking and Managing Non-Scale Victories

While the number on the scale is a common metric for tracking progress, it's essential to recognize that weight loss isn't the only measure of success. Non-scale

victories, such as improvements in energy levels, endurance, strength, and overall well-being, are equally important indicators of progress.

Keep a journal to track your fitness achievements, such as running longer distances, lifting heavier weights, or performing more repetitions in your workouts. Celebrate these accomplishments as they show that your body is making positive changes, even if the scale may not reflect it immediately.

26.8 The Importance of Sleep and Recovery in Weight Loss

Adequate sleep and recovery are often overlooked but play a significant role in weight loss and breaking through plateaus. Lack of sleep can disrupt hormones that regulate hunger and satiety, leading to increased cravings and overeating.

Strive for 7-9 hours of quality sleep each night to support weight loss efforts. Establish a consistent sleep schedule and create a calming bedtime routine to improve sleep quality.

In addition to sleep, recovery days are crucial for muscle repair and overall well-being. Overtraining can lead to stress on the body and hinder weight loss progress. Listen to your body and give it the rest it needs to recover fully.

26.9 Reframing Expectations and Celebrating Progress

It's essential to reframe your expectations and recognize that weight loss progress may not always be linear. Plateaus are a normal part of the weight loss journey, and they don't mean you're failing. Instead, see them as opportunities to learn more about your body and make necessary adjustments to continue progressing.

Celebrate every small victory, whether it's sticking to your healthy eating plan for a week, completing a challenging workout, or resisting temptation during a social gathering. Positive reinforcement can keep you motivated and focused on your ultimate weight loss goals.

26.10 Staying Motivated on Your Weight Loss Journey

Maintaining motivation throughout your weight loss journey is key to overcoming plateaus and achieving long-term success. Here are some tips to help you stay motivated:

1. Set Realistic Goals: Break your weight loss journey into smaller, achievable goals. Celebrate each milestone reached, no matter how small.

2. Visualize Success: Envision yourself achieving your weight loss goals and visualize the positive impact on your life.

3. Find a Support System: Surround yourself with supportive friends, family, or a weight loss group. Sharing your journey with others can provide encouragement and accountability.

4. Track Progress: Keep a food journal, track your workouts, and take progress photos to see how far you've come.

5. Reward Yourself: Treat yourself with non-food rewards when you achieve your goals. It could be a spa day, a new workout outfit, or a day off to relax.

6. Stay Positive: Focus on the positive changes you're making in your life, rather than dwelling on temporary setbacks.

7. Embrace Change: Be open to trying new foods, exercises, and approaches to your weight loss journey. Embracing change can lead to new breakthroughs.

Conclusion:

Breaking through weight loss plateaus requires a combination of nutritional strategies, exercise, and mindset adjustments. Understand that plateaus are a normal part of the weight loss process and stay committed to your goals. Reassess your nutrition, incorporate HIIT workouts, diversify your exercise routine, and prioritize sleep and recovery. Celebrate non-scale victories and stay positive throughout your journey. With determination and a proactive approach, you can overcome plateaus and continue progressing towards your weight loss goals.

Chapter 27: Nutritional Strategies for Sustainable Weight Maintenance

Weight loss is an achievement worth celebrating, but the real challenge lies in maintaining that weight loss over the long term. Sustainable weight maintenance requires a comprehensive approach that goes beyond diet and exercise. In this chapter, we will explore essential nutritional strategies for achieving and sustaining weight maintenance successfully.

27.1 Transitioning from Weight Loss to Weight Maintenance

Transitioning from weight loss to weight maintenance is a critical phase that requires a shift in mindset and lifestyle. During weight loss, the body undergoes changes in metabolism, hormone levels, and hunger signals. As you reach your goal weight, it's essential to recognize that the process does not end here. Instead, it's the beginning of a new chapter focused on maintaining your hard-earned progress.

27.2 Understanding the Role of Metabolic Adaptation

Metabolic adaptation is the body's natural response to changes in calorie intake and energy expenditure. As you lose weight, your body may adapt to the reduced calorie intake by lowering its resting metabolic rate (RMR). This reduction in RMR can slow down weight loss and make it challenging to continue losing weight at the same rate. Understanding metabolic adaptation can help set realistic expectations during weight maintenance and prevent feelings of frustration.

27.3 The Importance of Finding Your Maintenance Calories

Finding your maintenance calories is a crucial step in weight maintenance. These are the number of calories you need to consume to maintain your current weight. Calculating maintenance calories involves considering factors such as age, weight, height, activity level, and body composition. Online calculators or consultations with registered dietitians can help determine your maintenance calorie needs.

27.4 Balancing Food Choices for Long-Term Success

Balancing food choices is essential for sustainable weight maintenance. Focus on nutrient-dense foods, including fruits, vegetables, whole grains, lean proteins, and healthy fats. These foods provide essential nutrients while satisfying hunger and promoting overall health. Avoid excessive consumption of processed and sugary foods, as they can hinder progress and lead to weight regain.

27.5 Incorporating Regular Physical Activity into Your Routine

Regular physical activity is a cornerstone of weight maintenance. Engaging in both cardiovascular exercises and strength training helps preserve lean muscle mass, which aids in maintaining a higher metabolic rate. Aim for at least 150 minutes of moderate-intensity aerobic activity or 75 minutes of vigorous-intensity aerobic activity per week, along with muscle-strengthening activities on two or more days per week.

27.6 Mindful Eating for Continued Success

Mindful eating involves being present and aware of the eating experience. It helps individuals recognize hunger and fullness cues, preventing overeating and mindless snacking. Practicing mindful eating involves savoring the taste, texture, and satisfaction of food, avoiding distractions while eating, and eating slowly to allow the body to recognize fullness.

27.7 Building a Supportive Environment for Weight Maintenance

Building a supportive environment is essential for successful weight maintenance. Surround yourself with individuals who understand and support your weight maintenance goals. Engage in activities that promote a positive mindset and well-being, as emotional support can enhance long-term success.

27.8 Developing Healthy Habits for Life

Sustainable weight maintenance requires the development of healthy habits. Focus on building a routine that includes regular physical activity, balanced meals, and mindful eating. Make healthy choices a part of your daily life, as small consistent changes can lead to lasting results.

27.9 Monitoring Progress and Staying Accountable

Monitoring progress and staying accountable are vital for weight maintenance. Regularly track your weight, physical activity, and dietary choices to identify any changes or patterns. Consider seeking support from a registered dietitian or a weight management group to help with accountability.

27.10 Navigating Challenges and Bumps in the Road

Weight maintenance may come with challenges and setbacks. It's essential to recognize that bumps in the road are normal. Instead of getting discouraged, view these challenges as opportunities to learn and improve. Developing resilience and problem-solving skills can help navigate the obstacles that come with weight maintenance.

Chapter 28: Nutrition for Building Lean Muscle Mass

Building lean muscle mass requires a combination of proper nutrition, exercise, and recovery. In this chapter, we will delve into the essential role of nutrition in muscle growth and explore effective strategies for maximizing muscle development.

Chapter 28: Nutrition for Building Lean Muscle Mass

Building lean muscle mass requires a combination of proper nutrition, exercise, and recovery. In this chapter, we will delve into the essential role of nutrition in muscle growth and explore effective strategies for maximizing muscle development.

28.1 The Relationship Between Nutrition and Muscle Growth

Nutrition plays a pivotal role in muscle growth and development. To build lean muscle mass, it is crucial to consume an adequate amount of calories and nutrients that support muscle protein synthesis. Adequate protein intake, along with the right balance of carbohydrates and fats, provides the necessary fuel for muscle growth.

28.2 The Role of Protein in Muscle Synthesis

Protein is the primary macronutrient responsible for muscle synthesis. During strength training and exercise, muscle fibers undergo microscopic damage. Consuming protein-rich foods helps repair and rebuild these damaged muscle fibers, resulting in muscle growth over time. High-quality protein sources include lean meats, poultry, fish, eggs, dairy, legumes, and plant-based sources like tofu and tempeh.

28.3 Amino Acids and Their Impact on Muscle Repair

Amino acids are the building blocks of protein and play a vital role in muscle repair and growth. Essential amino acids cannot be produced by the body and must be obtained through diet. Consuming a variety of protein sources ensures you get all the essential amino acids needed for optimal muscle repair.

28.4 Proper Hydration for Muscle Function

Staying properly hydrated is critical for muscle function and growth. Dehydration can lead to decreased exercise performance and hinder muscle recovery. Aim to drink plenty of water throughout the day, and consider hydrating with electrolyte-rich beverages, especially during intense workouts.

28.5 Carbohydrates and Their Role in Muscle Energy

Carbohydrates provide the primary source of energy for muscle contractions during exercise. Consuming an adequate amount of carbohydrates before and after workouts ensures that muscles have enough glycogen stores to support energy demands. Focus on consuming complex carbohydrates from whole grains, fruits, and vegetables for sustained energy levels.

28.6 The Importance of Nutrient Timing for Muscle Building

Nutrient timing refers to the strategic consumption of nutrients around workouts to maximize muscle growth and recovery. Consuming protein and carbohydrates within an hour after exercise enhances muscle protein synthesis and glycogen replenishment. Pre-workout meals should include easily digestible carbohydrates for immediate energy.

28.7 Incorporating Strength Training into Your Routine

Strength training is a fundamental aspect of building lean muscle mass. Resistance exercises like weightlifting, bodyweight exercises, and resistance band workouts stimulate muscle fibers, leading to increased muscle size and strength. Include a variety of exercises that target different muscle groups for balanced muscle development.

28.8 Recovering with the Right Post-Workout Nutrition

Post-workout nutrition is essential for muscle recovery and growth. Consuming a balanced meal that includes protein and carbohydrates helps repair muscle fibers and replenish glycogen stores. Additionally, consider incorporating branched-chain amino acid (BCAA) supplements to support muscle recovery.

28.9 Balancing Muscle Gain with Body Composition Goals

Building lean muscle mass involves finding a balance between muscle gain and body composition goals. Some individuals may aim for significant muscle growth, while others may focus on gaining lean muscle while reducing body fat. Adjusting calorie intake and nutrient ratios based on individual goals is crucial for achieving the desired outcome.

28.10 Nutrition Strategies for Different Fitness Levels

Nutrition strategies for building lean muscle mass can vary based on individual fitness levels. Beginners may focus on establishing a foundation of proper nutrition and gradually increasing resistance training intensity. Intermediate and advanced individuals may incorporate periodization and advanced nutrition techniques to promote continuous muscle growth and prevent plateaus.

Chapter 29: Nutrition for Managing Cravings and Emotional Eating

In today's fast-paced world, managing food cravings and emotional eating can be a challenging task. In this chapter, we will explore the various aspects of cravings and emotional eating and discuss effective nutritional strategies to overcome these challenges.

29.1 Understanding Food Cravings and Emotional Eating

Food cravings are intense desires for specific foods, often high in sugar, fat, or salt. These cravings can be triggered by various factors, including stress, emotions, hormones, and even nutrient deficiencies. Emotional eating, on the other hand, refers to the consumption of food in response to emotions such as stress, sadness, boredom, or happiness, rather than actual hunger.

Understanding the root causes of food cravings and emotional eating is essential for implementing effective strategies to manage them.

29.2 The Link Between Cravings and Nutritional Deficiencies

In some cases, food cravings can be a signal that the body is lacking certain nutrients. For example, cravings for chocolate may indicate a need for magnesium, while cravings for salty foods could be related to low levels of sodium or other minerals.

It is essential to listen to our bodies and pay attention to the types of foods we crave. Addressing nutritional deficiencies through a balanced and varied diet can help reduce the intensity of cravings.

29.3 Mindful Eating Techniques for Curbing Cravings

Practicing mindful eating can be a powerful tool for curbing cravings and emotional eating. Mindful eating involves paying full attention to the eating experience, being present in the moment, and savoring each bite. By being mindful, we become more aware of our hunger and satiety cues, helping us distinguish between physical hunger and emotional cravings.

To practice mindful eating, try to eat slowly, chew your food thoroughly, and avoid distractions like TV or smartphones during meals.

29.4 Identifying Triggers for Emotional Eating

Understanding the triggers for emotional eating is crucial for breaking the cycle. Keep a food journal to track your emotions, eating patterns, and the specific triggers that lead to emotional eating episodes. Common triggers may include stress, boredom, loneliness, anxiety, or even certain social situations.

By identifying these triggers, you can develop alternative coping mechanisms to manage emotions without turning to food.

29.5 Coping Mechanisms for Dealing with Emotional Cravings

Instead of turning to food as a coping mechanism, explore alternative strategies to manage emotions. Engaging in physical activities like walking, yoga, or meditation can help reduce stress and emotional eating tendencies. Connecting with friends or loved ones for support, engaging in creative hobbies, or practicing deep breathing exercises can also provide healthy outlets for managing emotions.

Finding what works best for you and implementing these coping mechanisms can help break the emotional eating cycle.

29.6 The Impact of Stress on Cravings and Eating Habits

Stress can significantly influence cravings and eating habits. During periods of stress, the body releases hormones like cortisol, which can increase appetite and lead to cravings for high-calorie comfort foods.

Recognizing the connection between stress and food choices is essential for developing healthier stress-management techniques.

Regular exercise, relaxation techniques, and self-care practices can help alleviate stress and reduce the impact of stress on eating habits.

29.7 Satisfying Cravings with Healthy Substitutes

While it's essential to address the root causes of cravings, sometimes giving in to them in a healthier way can help prevent overindulgence. Instead of reaching for unhealthy snacks, consider healthier substitutes that satisfy the craving while providing valuable nutrients.

For example, if you're craving something sweet, opt for a piece of fruit or a small serving of dark chocolate. If you crave salty snacks, try air-popped popcorn or roasted chickpeas instead of chips.

29.8 Building a Support System for Overcoming Cravings

Having a supportive network can make a significant difference in managing cravings and emotional eating. Share your goals and challenges with friends, family members, or a support group. Surrounding yourself with people who understand your journey and can offer encouragement can help you stay motivated and accountable.

Consider seeking the guidance of a registered dietitian or a mental health professional experienced in disordered eating and emotional eating patterns.

29.9 Mindful Snacking and Portion Control

Mindful snacking and portion control are vital for managing cravings and emotional eating. Instead of mindlessly grabbing snacks when you feel a craving, take a moment to assess your hunger level. If you determine that you're physically hungry, choose a balanced snack that aligns with your nutritional goals.

Practice portion control by using smaller plates and bowls to help avoid overeating. Additionally, pre-portioning snacks into individual servings can prevent mindless eating and promote healthier habits.

29.10 Celebrating Progress and Success in Managing Cravings

Managing cravings and emotional eating is a journey that may have its ups and downs. Celebrate your progress and success, no matter how small it may seem. Acknowledge your efforts to make healthier choices and be kind to yourself during times of setbacks.

Remember that everyone faces challenges, and the key is to continue learning from experiences and striving for positive changes in your relationship with food and emotions.

Chapter 30: Nutrition for Energy and Vitality

In today's fast-paced world, maintaining high energy levels and vitality is essential for overall well-being and productivity. Proper nutrition plays a significant role in supporting energy production and sustaining vitality throughout the day. In this chapter, we will explore the various aspects of nutrition that contribute to energy and vitality.

30.1 Understanding the Role of Nutrients in Energy Production

Energy production in the body is a complex process that relies on the availability of essential nutrients. The macronutrients, including carbohydrates, proteins, and fats, are the primary sources of energy. Carbohydrates are the body's preferred energy source, providing a quick and readily available fuel for muscles and brain function. Proteins also contribute to energy production when carbohydrates are limited, while fats serve as a long-term energy reserve.

In addition to macronutrients, micronutrients like vitamins and minerals play crucial roles in energy metabolism. B-vitamins, in particular, are essential for converting food into energy and supporting overall metabolic processes.

30.2 Balancing Macronutrients for Sustained Energy

Balancing macronutrients is essential for sustained energy levels throughout the day. While carbohydrates provide quick energy, they should be balanced with proteins and fats to create a steady and lasting energy supply. Including a mix of complex carbohydrates, lean proteins, and healthy fats in each meal can help prevent energy crashes and promote stable blood sugar levels.

30.3 The Impact of Hydration on Energy Levels

Staying hydrated is vital for maintaining energy levels and overall well-being. Dehydration can lead to fatigue, decreased cognitive function, and reduced physical performance. Drinking an adequate amount of water throughout the day helps support proper digestion, nutrient absorption, and cellular function, all of which contribute to sustained energy.

30.4 Foods for Sustainable Energy Release

Choosing foods that promote sustainable energy release is crucial for maintaining vitality. Whole grains, such as brown rice, quinoa, and oats, provide a steady supply of complex carbohydrates and fiber, which slow down digestion and help regulate blood sugar levels.

Additionally, foods rich in protein, such as lean meats, poultry, fish, legumes, and nuts, contribute to prolonged energy release.

30.5 The Importance of B-Vitamins in Energy Metabolism

B-vitamins play a central role in energy metabolism. Thiamin (B1), riboflavin (B2), niacin (B3), pantothenic acid (B5), and pyridoxine (B6) are involved in converting carbohydrates, proteins, and fats into energy. Vitamin B12 and folic acid (B9) are also essential for red blood cell production and proper nerve function, contributing indirectly to energy levels.

Eating a varied diet that includes sources of B-vitamins, such as whole grains, legumes, nuts, seeds, leafy greens, and animal products, can help support optimal energy metabolism.

30.6 Managing Energy Crashes and Fatigue

Energy crashes and fatigue can occur due to various factors, including blood sugar fluctuations, nutrient deficiencies, inadequate sleep, and excessive stress. To manage energy crashes and fatigue, focus on balanced meals that include a mix of nutrients, avoid excessive consumption of sugary and processed foods, and prioritize restful sleep and stress management techniques.

30.7 The Role of Caffeine and Other Stimulants

Caffeine and other stimulants can provide a temporary boost in energy and alertness. However, relying on these substances for long-term energy can lead to dependence and disrupt natural energy rhythms. Moderate consumption of caffeine can be part of a healthy diet, but it's essential to avoid excessive intake and consider other lifestyle habits that promote sustained energy.

30.8 Creating Balanced Meals for Optimal Energy

Creating balanced meals is essential for supporting optimal energy levels. Incorporate a variety of nutrient-dense foods, including fruits, vegetables, whole grains, lean proteins, and healthy fats. Aim to include all major food groups in each meal, focusing on whole, minimally processed foods that provide sustained energy and essential nutrients.

30.9 The Connection Between Sleep and Energy Levels

Sleep is a fundamental aspect of energy and vitality. During sleep, the body undergoes essential restorative processes, and lack of sufficient sleep can lead to fatigue and decreased cognitive function. Establishing a regular sleep schedule, creating a relaxing bedtime routine, and ensuring a comfortable sleep environment are essential for promoting restful sleep and maintaining energy levels.

30.10 Lifestyle Habits for Boosting Energy and Vitality

In addition to nutrition, several lifestyle habits can enhance energy and vitality:

Regular Exercise: Engaging in regular physical activity improves circulation, oxygenates tissues, and increases endorphin levels, contributing to higher energy levels.

Stress Management: Chronic stress can deplete energy reserves and negatively impact overall well-being. Practicing stress-reduction techniques such as mindfulness, meditation, and deep breathing can help maintain vitality.

Time Management: Organizing daily tasks and setting priorities can reduce stress and create a more balanced and energized lifestyle.

Social Connection: Spending time with loved ones and engaging in social activities can boost mood and energy levels.

Getting Sunlight: Exposure to natural sunlight supports circadian rhythms and can positively impact energy and mood.

Conclusion:

Nutrition plays a pivotal role in supporting sustained energy and vitality. Balancing macronutrients, staying hydrated, and consuming nutrient-dense foods are essential for maintaining optimal energy levels throughout the day. Additionally, supporting energy metabolism through B-vitamins and adopting healthy lifestyle habits can further enhance overall vitality and well-being.

Chapter 31: Nutrition for a Healthy Gut-Brain Axis

The gut-brain axis is a bidirectional communication network between the gastrointestinal system and the brain. This intricate connection influences various physiological processes, including digestion, mood regulation, cognitive function, and even behavior. In recent years, researchers have uncovered the vital role of nutrition in supporting a healthy gut-brain axis. This chapter delves into the relationship between nutrition and the gut-brain axis, exploring the impact of different foods on gut health, mood, cognitive function, and overall mental well-being.

31.1 Understanding the Gut-Brain Connection

The gut and the brain are intricately linked through a complex network of nerves, hormones, and signaling molecules. The gut contains millions of neurons that communicate with the brain through the vagus nerve and other pathways. This communication allows the gut to influence brain function and vice versa. Additionally, the gut is home to trillions of beneficial bacteria known as the gut microbiota, which play a crucial role in the gut-brain axis.

31.2 The Role of the Microbiome in Brain Health

The gut microbiome refers to the diverse community of microorganisms residing in the gastrointestinal tract. These microorganisms, including bacteria, fungi, and viruses, have a profound impact on gut health and contribute to the gut-brain axis. The gut microbiome influences various aspects of brain function, such as neurotransmitter production, inflammation regulation, and the gut's permeability.

31.3 Foods that Support Gut-Brain Communication

Certain foods promote a healthy gut-brain axis by nourishing the gut microbiota and supporting gut health. Foods rich in prebiotics, such as garlic, onions, bananas, and oats, provide fuel for beneficial gut bacteria to thrive. Additionally, fermented foods like yogurt, sauerkraut, and kimchi contain probiotics that introduce beneficial live bacteria to the gut.

31.4 Gut Health and Its Influence on Mood

The gut-brain axis has a significant influence on mood regulation. The gut produces neurotransmitters like serotonin, often referred to as the "happy hormone," which plays a vital role in mood stabilization and emotional well-being. A healthy gut microbiome can contribute to optimal serotonin production, positively impacting mood and reducing the risk of mood disorders.

31.5 Nutrition for Improved Cognitive Function

Nutrition plays a critical role in supporting cognitive function. Consuming a diet rich in antioxidants, healthy fats, and essential nutrients can promote brain health and cognitive performance. Foods such as blueberries, avocados, fatty fish, and nuts are particularly beneficial for brain health due to their anti-inflammatory and neuroprotective properties.

31.6 The Impact of Gut Health on Mental Health

The gut-brain axis's dysfunction has been linked to various mental health conditions, including anxiety, depression, and stress-related disorders. An imbalanced gut microbiome and increased gut permeability can lead to systemic inflammation and disrupt the communication between the gut and the brain, affecting mood and mental well-being.

31.7 Probiotics and Their Potential Role in Brain Health

Probiotics, the beneficial live bacteria found in fermented foods and supplements, have shown promise in supporting brain health. These probiotics can positively influence gut microbiota composition, reduce inflammation, and improve neurotransmitter function, contributing to improved mental well-being.

31.8 The Gut-Brain Axis and Stress Management

The gut-brain axis plays a crucial role in the body's stress response. Chronic stress can disrupt gut microbiota balance and increase gut permeability, leading to gastrointestinal disturbances. In turn, gut imbalances can contribute to heightened stress responses and mood disturbances. Nurturing the gut-brain axis through nutrition can help improve the body's stress response and promote resilience to stress.

31.9 Nurturing the Gut-Brain Axis with Proper Nutrition

Maintaining a healthy gut-brain axis requires adopting a balanced and diverse diet that supports gut health. This includes consuming a variety of fruits, vegetables, whole grains, lean proteins, and healthy fats. Additionally, avoiding excessive consumption of processed and sugary foods can help maintain gut health and support the gut-brain connection.

31.10 Lifestyle Habits for Enhancing the Gut-Brain Connection

In addition to nutrition, certain lifestyle habits can enhance the gut-brain axis:

- Regular Exercise: Physical activity has been linked to improved gut health and cognitive function. Engaging in regular exercise can promote a healthy gut microbiome and support overall brain health.

- Stress Reduction: Managing stress through relaxation techniques, meditation, or mindfulness practices can positively impact the gut-brain axis and support mental well-being.

- Quality Sleep: Prioritizing restful sleep is essential for the gut-brain axis and overall health. Sufficient sleep allows the body to repair and restore, including gut health.

Conclusion:

The gut-brain axis is a fascinating and intricate connection that underscores the importance of nutrition for both gut health and brain function. Nourishing the gut with a balanced and diverse diet, including probiotic and prebiotic-rich foods, can positively influence mood, cognitive function, and overall mental well-being. By adopting healthy lifestyle habits and paying attention to gut health, individuals can enhance the gut-brain axis and support their overall health   and   vitality.

Chapter 32: Nutrition for a Healthy Thyroid Gland

The thyroid gland is a small, butterfly-shaped gland located in the front of the neck. Despite its size, the thyroid plays a crucial role in regulating various physiological processes throughout the body. Thyroid hormones are essential for metabolism, growth, development, and overall energy production. This chapter explores the vital role of nutrition in supporting a healthy thyroid gland and how dietary choices can impact thyroid function positively or negatively.

32.1 Understanding the Thyroid Gland and Its Function

The thyroid gland is responsible for producing two main hormones: triiodothyronine (T3) and thyroxine (T4). These hormones are synthesized from iodine and the amino acid tyrosine. Once released into the bloodstream, T3 and T4 travel throughout the body, influencing metabolism, body temperature, heart rate, and other vital functions.

The hypothalamus and pituitary gland play a crucial role in regulating thyroid hormone production. The hypothalamus releases thyrotropin-releasing hormone (TRH), which signals the pituitary gland to release thyroid-stimulating hormone (TSH). TSH, in turn, stimulates the thyroid gland to produce and release T3 and T4.

32.2 The Impact of Nutrition on Thyroid Hormones

Nutrition plays a pivotal role in maintaining proper thyroid function and ensuring the synthesis of adequate thyroid hormones. Adequate intake of essential nutrients, particularly iodine and selenium, is essential for the production of T3 and T4.

32.3 Iodine and Its Role in Thyroid Health

Iodine is a vital micronutrient required for the synthesis of thyroid hormones. The thyroid gland actively takes up iodine from the bloodstream to produce T3 and T4. Iodine deficiency can lead to thyroid disorders, including goiter and hypothyroidism.

Good dietary sources of iodine include iodized salt, seaweed, fish, and dairy products. In regions where iodine deficiency is prevalent, iodized salt and other iodine-fortified foods play a crucial role in preventing thyroid-related health issues.

32.4 Selenium and Its Importance for the Thyroid

Selenium is an essential trace mineral that plays a vital role in thyroid hormone metabolism. It is a key component of several enzymes involved in the conversion of T4 to the more active T3 form. Selenium deficiency can impair thyroid hormone production and conversion, leading to thyroid dysfunction.

Selenium-rich foods include Brazil nuts, seafood, organ meats, and whole grains. Ensuring adequate selenium intake can support optimal thyroid function and may reduce the risk of thyroid-related conditions.

32.5 Foods that Support Thyroid Function

Several other nutrients and foods support healthy thyroid function:

- Zinc: This trace mineral is involved in thyroid hormone production and plays a role in regulating TSH levels.
    - Iron: Adequate iron levels are necessary for thyroid hormone synthesis.
    - Tyrosine: As an amino acid, tyrosine is a building block for thyroid hormones. Foods rich in tyrosine include dairy products, poultry, fish, and almonds.
    - Vitamin D: Some research suggests that vitamin D may play a role in regulating thyroid function.

A balanced diet that includes a variety of nutrient-rich foods can support overall thyroid health.

32.6 Managing Thyroid Disorders through Diet

For individuals with thyroid disorders, diet can play a supportive role in managing symptoms and optimizing thyroid function. In some cases, lifestyle modifications and specific dietary choices can complement medical treatment for thyroid conditions.

32.7 Nutritional Considerations for Hypothyroidism

Hypothyroidism is a condition where the thyroid gland does not produce enough thyroid hormones. While nutrition alone cannot cure hypothyroidism, certain dietary practices may help manage symptoms and support overall thyroid health:

- Iodine Intake: For individuals with hypothyroidism caused by iodine deficiency, increasing iodine intake through iodized salt or iodine-rich foods may be beneficial. However, it is essential to work with a healthcare professional to determine the appropriate dosage.

- Selenium Supplementation: Some studies suggest that selenium supplementation may improve thyroid function in individuals with autoimmune thyroid conditions, such as Hashimoto's thyroiditis.

- Goitrogenic Foods: Goitrogens are substances that can interfere with iodine uptake by the thyroid gland. Cruciferous vegetables like broccoli, cabbage, and kale are goitrogenic when consumed in large quantities. Cooking these vegetables can reduce their goitrogenic effects.

32.8 Foods to Avoid for Thyroid Health

While most foods are generally safe for individuals with a healthy thyroid, certain foods and substances may interfere with thyroid hormone production or absorption:

- Soy: Soy contains goitrogens and may inhibit thyroid hormone synthesis when consumed in excess. However, moderate soy consumption is unlikely to cause issues for individuals with a healthy thyroid.

- Excessive Iodine: Consuming too much iodine, especially in supplement form, can lead to thyroid dysfunction, particularly in individuals with underlying thyroid conditions.

32.9 The Role of Gluten in Thyroid Dysfunction

Some individuals with autoimmune thyroid conditions, such as Hashimoto's thyroiditis, may also have gluten sensitivity. In these cases, adopting a gluten-free diet may reduce inflammation and antibody levels, potentially improving thyroid function.

32.10 Working with Healthcare Professionals for Thyroid Management

Individuals with thyroid disorders should work closely with healthcare professionals, including endocrinologists and registered dietitians, to develop personalized treatment plans. These plans may include dietary interventions, medication, and lifestyle modifications tailored to each individual's specific needs.

Conclusion:

Proper nutrition plays a vital role in supporting a healthy thyroid gland and optimizing thyroid hormone production. Adequate intake of iodine, selenium, and other essential nutrients is crucial for maintaining thyroid function. For individuals with thyroid disorders, working with healthcare professionals to develop personalized treatment plans can help manage symptoms and improve overall thyroid health. As with any medical condition, seeking professional guidance and following evidence-based practices is essential for optimal outcomes.

Chapter 33: The Role of Sleep in Weight Management

In the quest for successful weight management, many people focus on diet and exercise while overlooking a critical factor: sleep. Sleep plays a crucial role in regulating various physiological processes, including appetite, metabolism, and energy balance. This chapter explores the intricate relationship between sleep and weight management, highlighting how sleep duration, quality, and timing can significantly impact appetite, food choices, and overall weight.

33.1 Understanding the Relationship Between Sleep and Weight

Numerous studies have established a link between sleep and weight management. The quality and duration of sleep can influence hunger hormones, food intake, and energy expenditure. Chronic sleep deprivation, in particular, is associated with an increased risk of weight gain and obesity.

Sleep deprivation affects two key hormones involved in appetite regulation: leptin and ghrelin. Leptin, produced by fat cells, signals fullness to the brain and suppresses appetite. Ghrelin, on the other hand, is produced in the stomach and stimulates appetite. When sleep-deprived, the body produces more ghrelin and less leptin, leading to increased feelings of hunger and reduced feelings of fullness.

33.2 The Impact of Sleep Deprivation on Hunger Hormones

A lack of sleep disrupts the delicate balance between hunger hormones, leading to an increase in appetite and a preference for calorie-dense, high-carbohydrate foods. Sleep-deprived individuals often report cravings for sugary and high-fat foods, making it challenging to maintain a healthy diet.

Moreover, sleep deprivation can affect the brain's reward centers, making unhealthy food choices more appealing. This combination of hormonal changes and altered brain function can contribute to overeating and weight gain.

33.3 Sleep Quality and Its Influence on Appetite

Sleep quality is just as important as sleep duration in weight management. Restorative, deep sleep is essential for overall health, including proper appetite regulation. Disrupted or poor-quality sleep can lead to imbalances in appetite hormones and an increased risk of overeating.

Individuals with sleep disorders, such as insomnia or sleep apnea, are more likely to experience weight gain due to the disruptions in appetite hormones and energy regulation caused by their sleep disturbances.

33.4 The Role of Circadian Rhythms in Weight Regulation

The body's internal clock, known as the circadian rhythm, influences various physiological processes, including sleep-wake cycles and metabolism. Disruption of circadian rhythms, such as irregular sleep schedules or shift work, can lead to dysregulation of hunger hormones and impaired metabolism.

Late-night eating, a common behavior among those with irregular sleep patterns, can also contribute to weight gain. The body's natural circadian rhythm prepares it for fasting and rest during the nighttime hours. Consuming large meals late at night disrupts this natural rhythm, potentially leading to weight gain over time.

33.5 Creating a Sleep-Friendly Environment

Creating a sleep-friendly environment can improve sleep quality and support weight management efforts. Consider the following tips to optimize your sleep environment:

1. Comfortable Bed and Bedding: Invest in a comfortable mattress and bedding that promote restful sleep.

2. Darkness: Keep the bedroom dark to enhance melatonin production, the hormone that promotes sleep.

3. Noise Reduction: Minimize noise disturbances with earplugs or white noise machines.

4. Temperature: Maintain a comfortable room temperature for better sleep.

5. Limit Electronics: Avoid using electronic devices with bright screens before bedtime, as the blue light can disrupt sleep patterns.

6. Declutter: Keep the bedroom clean and clutter-free to create a calming environment.

33.6 Establishing a Bedtime Routine for Improved Sleep

Establishing a consistent bedtime routine can signal the body that it's time to wind down and prepare for sleep. A calming routine can reduce stress and promote better sleep quality. Consider incorporating the following into your bedtime routine:

1. Relaxation Techniques: Practice relaxation techniques such as deep breathing or meditation to reduce stress and promote relaxation.

2. Reading: Read a book or engage in another calming activity to shift your focus away from screens and work-related stress.

3. Limit Stimulants: Avoid caffeine, nicotine, and other stimulants in the hours leading up to bedtime.

4. Consistent Sleep Schedule: Try to go to bed and wake up at the same time each day to regulate your body's internal clock.

5. Avoid Heavy Meals: Avoid heavy meals close to bedtime, as digestion can interfere with sleep.

33.7 The Connection Between Stress and Sleep

Stress and sleep are closely interconnected. High levels of stress can disrupt sleep patterns, leading to difficulty falling asleep or staying asleep. Chronic stress can trigger the release of cortisol, a hormone that can interfere with sleep and appetite regulation.

Finding effective ways to manage stress, such as through exercise, meditation, or seeking support from friends or professionals, can improve sleep quality and support weight management goals.

33.8 Nutrition for Better Sleep Quality

Dietary choices can influence sleep quality. Some nutrients can promote relaxation and better sleep, while others can disrupt sleep patterns. Consider the following dietary tips for better sleep quality:

1. Limit Caffeine: Avoid consuming caffeine in the afternoon and evening, as it can interfere with

sleep.

2. Magnesium-Rich Foods: Magnesium is a mineral that promotes relaxation. Include magnesium-rich foods like leafy greens, nuts, and seeds in your diet.

3. Tryptophan Sources: Tryptophan is an amino acid that can enhance sleep. Foods like turkey, chicken, and dairy products are good sources of tryptophan.

4. Melatonin-Containing Foods: Melatonin is a hormone that regulates sleep-wake cycles. Foods like cherries and kiwi naturally contain melatonin and may support better sleep.

5. Light Evening Snack: A light snack before bed, such as a small piece of fruit or a handful of nuts, can help stabilize blood sugar levels and prevent hunger disruptions during the night.

33.9 Exercise and Its Impact on Sleep

Regular physical activity can improve sleep quality and support weight management efforts. However, the timing of exercise can also affect sleep. Some individuals may find that vigorous exercise close to bedtime can make it challenging to fall asleep.

For most people, moderate-intensity exercise earlier in the day can help promote better sleep quality. Regular physical activity can also help reduce stress and anxiety, contributing to improved sleep.

33.10 Prioritizing Restful Sleep for Successful Weight Management

In conclusion, sleep plays a critical role in weight management and overall health. The relationship between sleep and weight is multifaceted, involving hunger hormones, appetite regulation, and metabolic function. Prioritizing restful, high-quality sleep, and adopting healthy sleep habits can support weight management goals and improve overall well-being. By understanding the interplay between sleep and weight, individuals can optimize their sleep patterns and achieve successful, sustainable weight management outcomes.

Chapter 34: Nutrition for Improving Metabolism

Metabolism plays a vital role in the body's energy production and utilization. It encompasses a complex series of chemical processes that convert the food we eat into the energy needed for various bodily functions. A well-functioning metabolism is essential for maintaining a healthy weight, supporting physical activity, and promoting overall well-being. However, various factors, including age, genetics, diet, and lifestyle, can influence metabolic rate. In this chapter, we will explore nutrition strategies to improve metabolism and enhance energy expenditure for better weight management and overall health.

34.1 Understanding Metabolism and Its Components

Metabolism refers to all the chemical processes that occur in the body to maintain life. It includes two primary components:

1. Anabolism: This involves the building of complex molecules from simpler ones. Anabolic processes require energy and contribute to the growth and repair of tissues.

2. Catabolism: This entails the breakdown of complex molecules into simpler ones, releasing energy in the process. Catabolic processes provide the energy needed for bodily functions, such as breathing, circulation, and digestion.

Together, these processes regulate the body's energy balance, ensuring that energy intake from food matches energy expenditure for various physiological functions and activities.

34.2 The Impact of Age and Genetics on Metabolic Rate

Metabolic rate refers to the number of calories the body burns at rest to maintain basic physiological functions. It is influenced by age, genetics, body composition, and hormonal factors.

Age: Metabolic rate tends to decline with age due to a decrease in lean muscle mass and hormonal changes. This decline can result in a reduction in daily energy expenditure.

Genetics: Some individuals may have a genetically higher or lower metabolic rate, which can influence how efficiently their bodies burn calories.

Body Composition: Muscle tissue requires more energy to maintain than fat tissue. Therefore, individuals with higher muscle mass generally have a higher resting metabolic rate.

Hormones: Hormonal imbalances, such as thyroid dysfunction or insulin resistance, can affect metabolic rate.

While age and genetics play a role in metabolic rate, lifestyle factors, particularly diet and exercise, also significantly impact metabolism.

34.3 Factors Affecting Basal Metabolic Rate (BMR)

Basal Metabolic Rate (BMR) is the number of calories the body needs to maintain basic functions while at rest. Several factors influence BMR:

Body Size: Larger individuals generally have a higher BMR due to their greater body mass and higher energy requirements.

Body Composition: As mentioned earlier, individuals with higher muscle mass tend to have a higher BMR.

Age: BMR tends to decrease with age due to a decline in muscle mass and hormonal changes.

Gender: Men typically have a higher BMR than women, primarily due to their higher muscle mass.

Hormones: Thyroid hormones play a crucial role in regulating metabolism. An underactive thyroid can lead to a lower BMR.

Climate: Extreme temperatures can impact BMR as the body works harder to maintain its core temperature in hot or cold environments.

While some factors affecting BMR cannot be changed, such as age and genetics, others can be influenced through lifestyle choices, such as diet and exercise.

34.4 Boosting Metabolism through Proper Nutrition

Proper nutrition plays a significant role in supporting a healthy metabolism. By providing the body with the right nutrients and energy sources, you can optimize metabolic function and enhance energy expenditure.

Balanced Macronutrients: Consuming a balanced diet that includes carbohydrates, proteins, and fats in the right proportions is crucial for a well-functioning metabolism. Carbohydrates provide a readily available source of energy, while proteins support muscle mass and repair. Healthy fats are essential for hormone production and nutrient absorption.

Regular Meals and Snacks: Eating regular meals and snacks throughout the day helps maintain stable blood sugar levels, preventing energy fluctuations and supporting a consistent metabolic rate.

Avoiding Extreme Diets: Extremely low-calorie or restrictive diets can slow down metabolism as the body perceives a state of starvation and adapts by conserving energy.

Hydration: Staying hydrated is essential for metabolic processes to function optimally. Water is involved in digestion, nutrient transport, and waste removal.

34.5 The Role of Protein in Boosting Metabolism

Protein plays a crucial role in supporting a healthy metabolism. It has a high thermic effect, meaning that the body expends more energy to digest and process protein compared to carbohydrates and fats. This increased energy expenditure can contribute to an enhanced metabolic rate.

Moreover, protein is essential for building and maintaining lean muscle mass. Muscle tissue is metabolically active, meaning it requires more energy to maintain than fat tissue. By increasing protein intake and engaging in regular strength training, you can promote muscle growth and boost your metabolic rate.

Incorporate a variety of protein sources into your diet, such as lean meats, poultry, fish, eggs, dairy products, legumes, and plant-based protein sources like tofu and tempeh.

34.6 Thermic Effect of Food and Its Influence on Energy Expenditure

The thermic effect of food (TEF) refers to the energy expended during the digestion, absorption, and processing of nutrients in the diet. Different macronutrients have varying thermic effects:

Protein: As mentioned earlier, protein has

the highest thermic effect, with approximately 20-30% of its calories burned during digestion and processing.

Carbohydrates: Carbohydrates have a moderate thermic effect, with about 5-10% of their calories used during digestion.

Fats: Fats have the lowest thermic effect, with only about 0-3% of their calories expended during digestion.

By focusing on protein-rich foods and consuming a balanced diet that includes all three macronutrients, you can maximize the thermic effect of food and support a healthy metabolism.

34.7 The Impact of Physical Activity on Metabolism

Physical activity and exercise are essential factors for increasing energy expenditure and improving metabolic rate. Engaging in regular physical activity, such as cardio exercises, strength training, and high-intensity interval training (HIIT), can boost metabolism both during and after the workout.

Cardiovascular Exercise: Activities like running, cycling, and swimming can increase heart rate and calorie burn during the workout, leading to increased energy expenditure.

Strength Training: Lifting weights and performing resistance exercises help build and maintain muscle mass, which is metabolically active and contributes to a higher BMR.

High-Intensity Interval Training (HIIT): HIIT involves short bursts of intense exercise followed by brief periods of rest or lower-intensity exercise. This type of training can lead to an "afterburn" effect, where the body continues to burn calories at an elevated rate after the workout is completed.

Incorporate a mix of cardiovascular exercise, strength training, and HIIT into your fitness routine to maximize the impact on your metabolism.

34.8 Metabolism-Boosting Foods and Nutrients

Several foods and nutrients are believed to have metabolism-boosting properties, supporting weight management and overall health. While these foods alone won't drastically increase metabolism, incorporating them into a balanced diet can contribute to overall metabolic health.

Green Tea: Green tea contains catechins, a type of antioxidant that may support metabolism and fat oxidation.

Chili Peppers: Capsaicin, the compound responsible for the spicy taste in chili peppers, may temporarily boost metabolism and increase calorie expenditure.

Coffee: Caffeine, found in coffee, is a stimulant that can temporarily raise metabolic rate and enhance exercise performance.

Whole Grains: Whole grains, such as brown rice, quinoa, and oats, are complex carbohydrates that provide sustained energy and help stabilize blood sugar levels.

Iron-Rich Foods: Iron is essential for transporting oxygen throughout the body and supporting energy production. Include iron-rich foods like lean meats, spinach, and legumes in your diet.

34.9 Interval Training and Its Effect on Metabolism

Interval training, particularly High-Intensity Interval Training (HIIT), has gained popularity for its potential to boost metabolism and support weight loss efforts. HIIT involves alternating short bursts of high-intensity exercise with periods of lower-intensity exercise or rest. This pattern challenges the body, leading to increased calorie burn and improved metabolic rate.

The intensity and duration of HIIT workouts can be tailored to individual fitness levels. Beginners may start with shorter intervals and gradually increase the intensity and duration as they become more conditioned.

The afterburn effect, also known as excess post-exercise oxygen consumption (EPOC), is a key factor in HIIT's impact on metabolism. After a HIIT workout, the body requires additional oxygen to return to its pre-exercise state, leading to continued calorie burn for hours after the workout.

Incorporate HIIT workouts into your fitness routine, but be mindful of allowing adequate rest and recovery between sessions, as these workouts can be intense and place stress on the body.

34.10 Nurturing a Healthy Metabolism for Weight Management

To nurture a healthy metabolism and support weight management, consider the following lifestyle habits:

Regular Eating Schedule: Eat regular meals and snacks to maintain stable blood sugar levels and prevent energy crashes.

Stay Hydrated: Drink plenty of water throughout the day to support metabolic processes.

Balanced Diet: Consume a balanced diet that includes a mix of protein, carbohydrates, and healthy fats.

Strength Training: Include strength training exercises to build and maintain lean muscle mass.

Cardiovascular Exercise: Engage in regular cardio exercises to increase energy expenditure.

Interval Training: Incorporate HIIT or interval training to challenge your body and boost metabolism.

Adequate Sleep: Prioritize restful sleep to support overall health and metabolic function.

Reduce Stress: Manage stress through relaxation techniques like meditation or yoga.

Avoid Extreme Diets: Avoid extreme calorie restriction diets that can slow down metabolism.

Remember that everyone's metabolism is unique, and results may vary depending on individual factors. Sustainable weight management and improved metabolic health are achieved through a combination of proper nutrition, regular exercise, and positive lifestyle habits. Consult with a healthcare or nutrition professional to develop a personalized plan tailored to your specific needs and goals.

Chapter 35: Nutrition for Joint Health and Mobility

35.1 Understanding Joint Health and Nutrition

Joint health is crucial for maintaining mobility and overall quality of life. Joints are the connections between bones that allow for movement and flexibility. As we age or engage in repetitive activities, joint health can be compromised, leading to conditions such as osteoarthritis and reduced mobility.

Proper nutrition plays a significant role in supporting joint health. Certain nutrients have anti-inflammatory properties, help maintain joint cartilage, and reduce oxidative stress, all of which contribute to improved joint function. In this chapter, we will explore the importance of nutrition for joint health and mobility.

35.2 Anti-Inflammatory Foods for Joint Function

Chronic inflammation is associated with joint pain and deterioration. Including anti-inflammatory foods in your diet can help reduce inflammation and support joint function. Some anti-inflammatory foods include:

1. Fatty Fish: Fatty fish like salmon, mackerel, and sardines are rich in omega-3 fatty acids, which have potent anti-inflammatory properties.

2. Berries: Berries such as blueberries, strawberries, and cherries are packed with antioxidants that can help combat inflammation.

3. Leafy Greens: Vegetables like spinach, kale, and broccoli are rich in antioxidants and other anti-inflammatory compounds.

4. Turmeric: Turmeric contains curcumin, a compound known for its powerful anti-inflammatory effects.

5. Ginger: Ginger has anti-inflammatory properties and can help reduce joint pain and swelling.

6. Extra Virgin Olive Oil: Olive oil contains oleocanthal, which has been shown to have similar anti-inflammatory effects as ibuprofen.

Incorporating these foods into your diet can support joint health and reduce inflammation.

35.3 Omega-3 Fatty Acids and Their Impact on Joints

Omega-3 fatty acids, specifically eicosapentaenoic acid (EPA) and docosahexaenoic acid (DHA), are essential fats that play a vital role in reducing inflammation and supporting joint health. These fatty acids are abundant in fatty fish, such as salmon, mackerel, and trout.

The anti-inflammatory properties of omega-3s can help alleviate joint pain and stiffness, making them beneficial for individuals with conditions like osteoarthritis or rheumatoid arthritis. Omega-3s also support the lubrication of joints, promoting smooth movement and reducing wear and tear on cartilage.

For those who do not consume fish, plant-based sources of omega-3s include chia seeds, flaxseeds, and walnuts. Omega-3 supplements are also available, but it is essential to consult with a healthcare professional before starting any supplementation.

35.4 Foods Rich in Collagen for Joint Support

Collagen is the main structural protein in connective tissues, including joints and cartilage. Consuming foods rich in collagen can provide building blocks for joint support and promote overall joint health.

Bone Broth: Bone broth is made by simmering animal bones and connective tissues, releasing collagen, minerals, and other nutrients. Drinking bone broth or using it as a base for soups and stews can be beneficial for joint health.

Chicken Skin and Fish Scales: These parts of poultry and fish are rich in collagen and can be consumed when cooked.

Collagen Supplements: Collagen supplements are also available in various forms, including powders, capsules, and gummies. These supplements can be convenient for individuals who may not consume collagen-rich foods regularly.

While collagen supplementation can support joint health, it is essential to remember that a balanced diet with a variety of nutrients is crucial for overall well-being.

35.5 Hydration and Its Influence on Joint Mobility

Staying hydrated is essential for overall health, and it also plays a role in joint health and mobility. Water helps lubricate the joints, allowing for smooth movement and reducing friction between bones. Proper hydration can also help cushion the joints and support shock absorption during physical activities.

Dehydration can lead to joint stiffness and discomfort, making it important to drink an adequate amount of water throughout the day. The recommended daily water intake varies depending on individual factors such as age, gender, activity level, and climate.

In addition to water, consuming foods with high water content, such as fruits and vegetables, can contribute to hydration and support joint health.

35.6 The Role of Antioxidants in Reducing Joint Inflammation

Antioxidants are compounds that help neutralize harmful free radicals in the body, which can cause oxidative stress and inflammation. By reducing oxidative stress, antioxidants can help protect joint tissues and support overall joint health.

Vitamins A, C, and E, as well as selenium and zinc, are potent antioxidants found in various foods. Including a wide variety of fruits, vegetables, nuts, and seeds in your diet can provide a rich array of antioxidants.

Some specific antioxidants with anti-inflammatory properties include:

Vitamin C: Found in citrus fruits, strawberries, bell peppers, and broccoli, vitamin C can help reduce inflammation and support collagen synthesis.

Vitamin E: Found in nuts, seeds, and vegetable oils, vitamin E can help protect joint tissues from oxidative damage.

Selenium: Found in Brazil nuts, fish, and poultry, selenium has antioxidant properties that can support joint health.

Berries: Berries, such as blueberries and cherries, are rich in anthocyanins, a type of antioxidant that

can help reduce inflammation.

35.7 Maintaining a Healthy Weight for Joint Health

Maintaining a healthy weight is crucial for joint health, especially for weight-bearing joints such as the knees and hips. Excess body weight puts additional stress on the joints, leading to increased wear and tear on the cartilage and joint tissues.

Obesity is a significant risk factor for osteoarthritis, as the excess weight places strain on the joints and can accelerate joint degeneration. Losing weight through a combination of a balanced diet and regular physical activity can significantly reduce the burden on the joints and improve joint function.

Consult with a healthcare professional or a registered dietitian to develop a personalized weight management plan that aligns with your specific needs and goals.

35.8 Nutrition for Managing Arthritis Symptoms

Arthritis is a group of conditions that cause joint inflammation and pain. While proper nutrition cannot cure arthritis, certain dietary choices can help manage symptoms and improve overall joint health.

Omega-3 Fatty Acids: As mentioned earlier, omega-3 fatty acids have anti-inflammatory properties that can help reduce joint pain and inflammation.

Turmeric and Curcumin: Turmeric contains curcumin, a compound known for its anti-inflammatory effects. Adding turmeric to your diet or taking curcumin supplements may provide relief from arthritis symptoms for some individuals.

Ginger: Ginger has anti-inflammatory properties and may help reduce arthritis-related pain and stiffness.

Avoiding Trigger Foods: Some individuals with arthritis may experience increased symptoms after consuming certain foods, such as processed foods, sugary snacks, and foods high in saturated fats. Identifying trigger foods and reducing their intake may help manage symptoms.

Consulting with a healthcare professional or a registered dietitian is essential for individuals with arthritis to develop a nutrition plan that suits their specific needs and helps manage their symptoms effectively.

35.9 Exercise and Its Effect on Joint Function

While nutrition is a critical component of joint health, regular exercise is equally important. Exercise can help improve joint function, flexibility, and strength, reducing the risk of joint-related issues and supporting overall mobility.

Low-Impact Exercises: Low-impact exercises, such as walking, swimming, and cycling, are gentle on the joints and can help improve cardiovascular health without putting excessive stress on the joints.

Strength Training: Strength training exercises, using resistance bands or weights, can help strengthen the muscles surrounding the joints, providing better support and stability.

Flexibility Exercises: Stretching and flexibility exercises, like yoga and Pilates, can help improve joint range of motion and reduce stiffness.

A well-rounded exercise routine that includes a mix of cardiovascular, strength, and flexibility exercises can support joint health and mobility.

35.10 Creating a Nutritional Plan for Healthy Joints

To promote joint health and mobility, consider the following tips for creating a nutritional plan:

1. Eat a Balanced Diet: Consume a variety of nutrient-dense foods, including fruits, vegetables, whole grains, lean proteins, and healthy fats.

2. Include Omega-3 Fatty Acids: Incorporate fatty fish or plant-based sources of omega-3s, such as chia seeds and walnuts, into your diet.

3. Stay Hydrated: Drink plenty of water throughout the day to support joint lubrication and function.

4. Limit Inflammatory Foods: Minimize the intake of processed foods, sugary snacks, and foods high in saturated fats.

5. Add Collagen-Rich Foods: Consider including bone broth or collagen supplements to support joint health.

6. Maintain a Healthy Weight: If necessary, work towards achieving and maintaining a healthy weight to reduce joint stress.

7. Avoid Trigger Foods: Pay attention to how certain foods affect your joints and adjust your diet accordingly.

8. Work with Professionals: Consult with a registered dietitian or healthcare professional to create a personalized nutritional plan that aligns with your specific health needs and goals.

In conclusion, proper nutrition plays a critical role in supporting joint health and mobility. Including anti-inflammatory foods, omega-3 fatty acids, collagen-rich foods, and antioxidants in your diet can help reduce joint inflammation and provide essential nutrients for joint function. Maintaining a healthy weight and engaging in regular exercise further contribute to joint health. A well-balanced diet, combined with a healthy lifestyle, can lead to improved joint function and overall quality of life.

Chapter 36: Nutrition for Enhanced Athletic Performance

36.1 Optimizing Nutrition for Athletic Goals

Athletes, whether amateur or professional, rely on optimal nutrition to achieve their performance goals. Proper nutrition plays a crucial role in providing the necessary energy, nutrients, and hydration to support athletic performance, recovery, and overall well-being. In this chapter, we will explore the key aspects of nutrition for enhancing athletic performance.

To optimize nutrition for athletic goals, it is essential to consider individual factors such as age, gender, sport or activity type, training intensity, and competition schedule. A well-balanced diet that meets energy demands, provides essential nutrients, and supports recovery is fundamental for athletes.

36.2 Pre-Game and Pre-Workout Nutrition Strategies

Pre-game or pre-workout nutrition is vital to provide the body with adequate fuel and prepare for physical exertion. The goals of pre-game nutrition include optimizing energy levels, maintaining blood glucose levels, and reducing the risk of fatigue during exercise.

Carbohydrates are the primary source of energy for muscles during high-intensity activities. Consuming a carbohydrate-rich meal or snack before exercise can help top up glycogen stores and sustain energy levels. Examples of pre-game carbohydrate-rich foods include whole-grain bread, pasta, rice, fruits, and starchy vegetables.

Protein is also essential before exercise, as it helps support muscle repair and growth. Including a moderate amount of protein in the pre-game meal can be beneficial. Some protein sources include lean meats, poultry, fish, tofu, and dairy products.

It is essential to consider individual tolerance and digestion time when planning pre-game meals. Eating a large meal right before exercise may lead to discomfort, so some athletes prefer smaller meals or snacks closer to their training or competition time.

36.3 The Role of Carbohydrates in Endurance Performance

Endurance athletes, such as distance runners, cyclists, and swimmers, heavily rely on carbohydrates for prolonged exercise. Carbohydrates are stored in the form of glycogen in muscles and the liver, serving as a readily available energy source during endurance activities.

Carbohydrate intake before, during, and after endurance exercise is critical for maintaining blood glucose levels and delaying fatigue. Before long training sessions or competitions, athletes may benefit from consuming a carbohydrate-rich meal or snack to top up glycogen stores.

During prolonged exercise, consuming easily digestible carbohydrates, such as sports drinks, gels, or energy chews, can help maintain energy levels and delay fatigue. The recommended carbohydrate intake during endurance exercise ranges from 30 to 60 grams per hour, depending on individual factors and exercise intensity.

After endurance exercise, replenishing glycogen stores with carbohydrates is crucial for recovery. Including carbohydrates along with protein in the post-exercise meal or snack can help support muscle recovery and glycogen resynthesis.

36.4 Protein and Its Impact on Muscle Performance

Protein plays a significant role in muscle performance and recovery for athletes engaging in strength training and other high-intensity activities. During exercise, muscle fibers experience micro-tears, and adequate protein intake supports the repair and growth of these muscles.

The protein requirements for athletes vary depending on their training intensity, body composition goals, and sport type. Endurance athletes may require 1.2 to 1.4 grams of protein per kilogram of body weight per day, while strength athletes may need 1.4 to 2.0 grams per kilogram of body weight per day.

Good sources of protein for athletes include lean meats, poultry, fish, eggs, dairy products, tofu, legumes, and protein-rich plant-based foods.

36.5 Hydration and Electrolyte Balance for Athletic Performance

Proper hydration is essential for athletic performance and overall health. Dehydration can lead to decreased exercise performance, increased risk of heat-related illnesses, and impaired cognitive function.

The amount of fluid an athlete needs depends on various factors, including exercise intensity, duration, environmental conditions, and individual sweat rate. Monitoring body weight before and after exercise can provide insights into fluid loss and help determine fluid replacement needs.

Electrolytes, such as sodium, potassium, calcium, and magnesium, play a crucial role in fluid balance and nerve function. During prolonged exercise, especially in hot and humid conditions, athletes may lose significant amounts of electrolytes through sweat.

Sports drinks or electrolyte-replenishing beverages can be beneficial for athletes engaged in intense and prolonged exercise, as they help replace lost fluids and electrolytes. However, for shorter-duration and lower-intensity activities, water is usually sufficient for hydration needs.

36.6 Post-Workout Nutrition for Recovery and Muscle Repair

The post-workout period is a critical window for recovery and muscle repair. Consuming the right nutrients after exercise can help replenish glycogen stores, repair damaged muscles, and optimize recovery.

Carbohydrates are essential after exercise to restore glycogen levels in muscles and the liver. Including a mix of complex and simple carbohydrates in the post-workout meal or snack can be beneficial.

Protein is crucial for supporting muscle recovery and growth. Consuming protein after exercise can help repair muscle tissue damaged during training or competition. Aim to consume protein sources

Chapter 37: Nutrition for Healthy Aging and Weight Management

37.1 Understanding Age-Related Changes and Nutrition

Aging is a natural and inevitable process that brings about various physiological changes in the body. As we age, our nutritional needs and metabolism also change, and it becomes essential to adjust our diet to support healthy aging and weight management. In this chapter, we will explore the key aspects of nutrition for promoting healthy aging and managing weight effectively.

As we age, our body composition tends to shift, with a decline in muscle mass and an increase in body fat. This change in body composition can affect metabolism and energy expenditure. Additionally, age-related changes in hormones and organ function can impact how our body processes nutrients.

37.2 The Impact of Metabolic Slowdown with Age

One of the significant factors contributing to weight management challenges in older adults is metabolic slowdown. Metabolic rate, which refers to the number of calories the body burns at rest, tends to decrease with age. As a result, older individuals may find it harder to maintain their weight or lose weight through diet alone.

To counteract the effects of metabolic slowdown, it is crucial for older adults to engage in regular physical activity, including both cardiovascular exercises and strength training. Exercise can help boost metabolism, preserve muscle mass, and support weight management efforts.

37.3 Nutritional Considerations for Maintaining Muscle Mass

Preserving muscle mass is vital for healthy aging, as it helps maintain strength, mobility, and independence. Adequate protein intake becomes especially important for older adults to support muscle health and prevent age-related muscle loss, known as sarcopenia.

Including high-quality protein sources in the diet, such as lean meats, poultry, fish, eggs, dairy, legumes, and tofu, can help older adults meet their protein needs. Distributing protein intake evenly throughout the day, rather than consuming it all in one meal, may also enhance muscle protein synthesis.

37.4 Balancing Macronutrients for Aging Individuals

While the overall macronutrient needs for older adults are similar to those of younger adults, individual factors, such as activity level, health status, and metabolic changes, may influence the optimal macronutrient distribution.

Carbohydrates are an essential source of energy for older adults, but focusing on complex carbohydrates, such as whole grains, fruits, and vegetables, is recommended to support steady blood sugar levels and provide essential nutrients.

Fats are also crucial for older adults' health, particularly healthy fats like monounsaturated and polyunsaturated fats found in nuts, seeds, avocados, and olive oil. Limiting saturated and trans fats is essential for heart health.

37.5 The Role of Nutrients in Bone Health and Osteoporosis Prevention

Bone health becomes a significant concern as we age, as the risk of osteoporosis and fractures increases. Calcium and vitamin D are two crucial nutrients for maintaining strong and healthy bones.

A diet rich in calcium can be achieved through dairy products, leafy greens, fortified plant-based milk, and calcium-fortified foods. Vitamin D can be obtained from sunlight exposure and dietary sources like fatty fish, egg yolks, and fortified foods.

Other nutrients, such as magnesium, vitamin K, and zinc, also play a role in bone health and should be included in a well-rounded diet.

37.6 Hydration and Its Effect on Aging

Staying adequately hydrated is essential for people of all ages, but it becomes particularly crucial for older adults. As we age, the sensation of thirst may diminish, leading to inadequate fluid intake.

Proper hydration is essential for maintaining healthy kidney function, digestion, cognitive function, and temperature regulation. Drinking water regularly and consuming water-rich foods, like fruits and vegetables, can help older adults stay hydrated.

37.7 Nutritional Support for Cognitive Function and Memory

Cognitive decline is a common concern with aging, and proper nutrition can play a role in supporting brain health and cognitive function. Foods rich in antioxidants, such as fruits and vegetables, can help protect the brain from oxidative stress and inflammation.

Omega-3 fatty acids, found in fatty fish like salmon and mackerel, are crucial for brain health and may help support memory and cognitive function.

Additionally, maintaining stable blood sugar levels through a balanced diet can also promote brain health and reduce the risk of cognitive decline.

37.8 Addressing Age-Related Health Conditions through Diet

Certain age-related health conditions, such as hypertension, diabetes, and cardiovascular diseases, may require specific dietary modifications. For example, reducing sodium intake can help manage blood pressure, while controlling carbohydrate intake can support blood sugar management in individuals with diabetes.

Working with a healthcare professional or a registered dietitian can be beneficial in developing a personalized dietary plan to address specific health concerns and support overall well-being in older adults.

37.9 The Connection Between Sleep and Aging

Quality sleep is essential for overall health and well-being, and it becomes even more critical as we age. Many older adults may experience changes in sleep patterns, including difficulty falling asleep or staying asleep.

Certain dietary practices can support better sleep, such as avoiding large meals or heavy snacks close to bedtime and limiting caffeine and alcohol intake in the

evening. Creating a relaxing bedtime routine can also promote better sleep quality.

37.10 Aging Gracefully with a Healthy Diet and Lifestyle

In conclusion, nutrition plays a significant role in promoting healthy aging and managing weight effectively. Older adults can support their overall health and well-being by maintaining a balanced diet that meets their nutritional needs, staying physically active, staying hydrated, and getting adequate sleep.

Aging gracefully involves embracing healthy lifestyle habits that nourish the body and mind, helping older adults enjoy a high quality of life and independence as they age. By making mindful choices about nutrition and lifestyle, older adults can optimize their well-being and age with grace and vitality.

Chapter 38: Nutrition for Heart-Healthy Aging

As individuals age, maintaining cardiovascular health becomes increasingly important for overall well-being and quality of life. Nutrition plays a crucial role in preventing heart disease and supporting heart-healthy aging. In this chapter, we will explore the impact of aging on cardiovascular health, the role of nutrition in preventing heart disease, and specific nutrients and foods that promote heart health in the aging population.

38.1 The Impact of Aging on Cardiovascular Health

As people age, the cardiovascular system undergoes natural changes that can affect heart health. Blood vessels may become stiffer and less flexible, leading to increased blood pressure. The heart muscle may also weaken, reducing its pumping efficiency. These age-related changes can contribute to an increased risk of heart disease, including conditions such as hypertension, atherosclerosis, and heart failure.

While aging is a natural process, lifestyle factors, including nutrition and physical activity, can significantly influence cardiovascular health and reduce the risk of heart disease.

38.2 The Role of Nutrition in Preventing Heart Disease

A heart-healthy diet is a cornerstone of cardiovascular disease prevention, and it becomes even more critical as individuals age. Research has shown that a balanced diet, rich in nutrient-dense foods, can help reduce the risk of heart disease and promote heart-healthy aging.

The Mediterranean diet, characterized by abundant fruits, vegetables, whole grains, legumes, nuts, seeds, and olive oil, is one of the most well-researched dietary patterns for heart health. This diet is known for its anti-inflammatory properties and positive effects on cholesterol levels, blood pressure, and overall cardiovascular health.

38.3 Omega-3 Fatty Acids and Heart Health in Aging

Omega-3 fatty acids, particularly eicosapentaenoic acid (EPA) and docosahexaenoic acid (DHA), are essential fats with powerful cardiovascular benefits. These fatty acids are known to reduce inflammation, improve blood vessel function, and lower triglyceride levels. They may also help stabilize heart rhythm and decrease the risk of arrhythmias.

Fatty fish, such as salmon, mackerel, and sardines, are excellent sources of EPA and DHA. For those who do not consume fish regularly, supplementation with high-quality fish oil capsules may be considered after consulting with a healthcare professional.

38.4 Antioxidants for Cardiovascular Protection

Antioxidants play a crucial role in protecting the cardiovascular system from oxidative stress, which can contribute to the development of atherosclerosis and other heart conditions. Antioxidants neutralize free radicals, unstable molecules that can damage cells and tissues in the body.

Fruits and vegetables are rich sources of antioxidants, including vitamins C and E, beta-carotene, and flavonoids. Berries, citrus fruits, leafy greens, and colorful vegetables should be incorporated into the diet to boost antioxidant intake and support heart health.

38.5 Nutrients for Maintaining Healthy Blood Pressure

Hypertension, or high blood pressure, is a significant risk factor for heart disease and stroke. As individuals age, maintaining healthy blood pressure becomes increasingly important. Several nutrients can help regulate blood pressure and promote heart-healthy aging.

Potassium is a mineral that plays a key role in maintaining healthy blood pressure. It balances the effects of sodium, which can raise blood pressure, and supports proper muscle function, including the heart. Foods rich in potassium include bananas, sweet potatoes, spinach, and avocados.

Magnesium is another essential mineral that contributes to heart health and blood pressure regulation. Magnesium-rich foods include nuts, seeds, whole grains, and leafy greens.

38.6 Foods that Support Cholesterol Levels

High cholesterol levels, particularly elevated levels of LDL (low-density lipoprotein) cholesterol, are a significant risk factor for heart disease. Aging can sometimes lead to unfavorable changes in cholesterol levels, making it important to focus on foods that support healthy cholesterol levels.

Soluble fiber is known to help lower LDL cholesterol levels. Oats, barley, legumes, and fruits like apples and oranges are excellent sources of soluble fiber.

Nuts, particularly almonds and walnuts, have been shown to improve cholesterol profiles. They are rich in heart-healthy fats, fiber, and antioxidants.

Plant sterols and stanols are compounds found in certain plant foods that can help reduce LDL cholesterol absorption in the intestines. Foods fortified with plant sterols, such as some margarines and orange juice, can be incorporated into a heart-healthy diet.

38.7 Nutritional Strategies for Preventing Atherosclerosis

Atherosclerosis is a condition where plaque builds up inside the arteries, narrowing them and restricting blood flow. Preventing atherosclerosis is crucial for maintaining healthy blood vessels and reducing the risk of heart attacks and strokes.

A diet rich in fruits, vegetables, and whole grains provides essential nutrients and antioxidants that help prevent the formation of plaque. Additionally, limiting the intake of saturated and trans fats is essential, as these fats can contribute to the development of plaque in the arteries.

Incorporating regular physical activity into the daily routine can also support cardiovascular health and reduce the risk of atherosclerosis.

38.8 The Importance of Exercise in Heart-Healthy Aging

In addition to proper nutrition, regular physical activity is essential for heart-healthy aging. Exercise strengthens the heart muscle, improves blood flow, and helps maintain healthy blood pressure and cholesterol levels.

A combination of aerobic exercise, such as walking, swimming, or cycling, and strength training is ideal for supporting cardiovascular health. Exercise can also improve overall energy levels and quality of life in aging individuals.

38.9 Managing Age-Related Heart Conditions with Diet

As individuals age, they may be more susceptible to certain heart conditions, such as atrial fibrillation, heart failure, or valvular heart disease. Managing these conditions may require dietary modifications to support heart health and manage symptoms.

For example, those with heart failure may need to limit fluid intake and reduce sodium consumption to prevent fluid retention. Those with atrial fibrillation may need to avoid excessive caffeine and alcohol, as these substances can trigger irregular heart rhythms.

38.10 Creating a Heart-Healthy Meal Plan for Aging Adults

Designing a heart-healthy meal plan for aging adults involves a holistic approach that considers nutrient needs, health conditions, and individual preferences. Here are some general guidelines for creating a heart-healthy meal plan:

- Emphasize fruits and vegetables: Aim to fill half the plate with colorful fruits and vegetables. They are rich in vitamins, minerals, fiber, and antioxidants that support heart health.

- Choose whole grains: Opt for whole grains such as brown rice, quinoa, whole wheat bread, and oats. Whole grains provide sustained energy and promote heart health.

- Include lean proteins: Choose lean sources of protein, such as fish, poultry without the skin, legumes, and tofu. Limit red meat and processed meats, which are higher in saturated fats.

- Incorporate heart-healthy fats: Include sources of healthy fats in the diet, such as avocados, nuts, seeds, and olive oil. These fats support heart health and provide essential nutrients.

- Limit added sugars and salt: Minimize the consumption of sugary foods and beverages, as well as foods high in sodium. Excessive sugar and salt intake can negatively impact heart health.

- Hydration: Drink plenty of water throughout the day to stay hydrated and support cardiovascular function.

- Consider dietary supplements: In some cases, dietary supplements may be recommended to fill nutrient gaps or support specific heart health needs. However, it is essential to consult with a healthcare professional before starting any new supplements.

In conclusion, nutrition plays a vital role in promoting heart-healthy aging and reducing the risk of heart disease in older adults. A balanced and nutrient-rich diet, along with regular physical activity, can support cardiovascular health and enhance overall well-being. Additionally, managing age-related heart conditions may require dietary modifications tailored to individual health needs. Consulting with a registered dietitian or healthcare professional can provide

personalized guidance and support for maintaining heart health
throughout the aging process.

Chapter 39: Nutrition for Managing Menopause and Weight

Menopause is a natural and inevitable stage in a woman's life, marking the end of her reproductive years. It typically occurs in the late 40s or early 50s and is characterized by a significant decline in estrogen and other reproductive hormones. These hormonal changes can have various effects on the body, including metabolism, bone health, and weight management. Proper nutrition during menopause plays a vital role in managing symptoms, supporting overall health, and maintaining a healthy weight. In this chapter, we will explore the impact of menopause on weight and metabolism, the nutritional considerations for menopause symptoms, and the role of exercise and mindful eating in managing menopause-related weight changes.

39.1 Understanding Menopause and Its Impact on Weight

During menopause, the ovaries gradually stop producing estrogen and other hormones, leading to a variety of physical and emotional changes. Many women experience weight gain or changes in body composition during this time, particularly an increase in abdominal fat. These changes can be attributed to hormonal fluctuations, aging, lifestyle factors, and genetics.

Estrogen, in particular, plays a role in regulating body fat distribution. As estrogen levels decrease, fat tends to redistribute from the hips and thighs to the abdomen. This visceral fat, also known as belly fat, is metabolically active and can increase the risk of cardiovascular disease and other health issues.

It is essential to note that not all women will experience weight gain during menopause. Individual factors such as genetics, lifestyle, and pre-menopausal weight can influence weight changes during this transition.

39.2 Hormonal Changes and Their Influence on Metabolism

The hormonal changes that occur during menopause can also affect metabolism. Estrogen plays a role in regulating metabolic rate, and its decline can lead to a slower metabolism. A slower metabolism means that the body burns fewer calories at rest, making it easier to gain weight.

In addition to estrogen, other hormones like progesterone and testosterone also fluctuate during menopause, further impacting metabolism and body composition.

39.3 Nutritional Considerations for Menopause Symptoms

Proper nutrition during menopause is crucial for managing symptoms and promoting overall well-being. Some common menopause symptoms that can be influenced by diet include:

- Hot flashes: Certain foods and beverages, such as spicy foods, caffeine, and alcohol, may trigger hot flashes in some women. Reducing or avoiding these triggers can help manage hot flashes.

- Mood swings: Nutrient-rich foods that support brain health, such as omega-3 fatty acids and B-vitamins, may help stabilize mood and reduce irritability.

- Fatigue: A balanced diet that provides adequate energy and nutrients can help combat fatigue and support energy levels.

- Sleep disturbances: Limiting caffeine and adopting a regular sleep schedule can improve sleep quality during menopause.

39.4 Foods for Balancing Hormones during Menopause

Certain foods can help balance hormones and support overall hormonal health during menopause:

- Flaxseeds and chia seeds: These seeds are rich in lignans, which are phytoestrogens that may help balance hormone levels in the body.

- Soy products: Soy contains isoflavones, another type of phytoestrogen that may have estrogen-like effects in the body.

- Fruits and vegetables: Colorful fruits and vegetables are rich in antioxidants, vitamins, and minerals that support hormonal health and reduce inflammation.

- Healthy fats: Consuming sources of healthy fats, such as avocados, nuts, and olive oil, can help support hormone production and reduce inflammation.

39.5 The Role of Phytoestrogens in Menopause Management

Phytoestrogens are plant compounds that have a similar structure to estrogen and can bind to estrogen receptors in the body. They are found in various plant-based foods, including soy products, flaxseeds, sesame seeds, and legumes.

During menopause, when estrogen levels decline, phytoestrogens may help alleviate menopausal symptoms by providing a mild estrogenic effect. They can also help regulate hormone balance and support bone health.

It is essential to consume phytoestrogens as part of a balanced diet and not as a substitute for medical treatment or hormone therapy. As with any dietary changes, it is recommended to consult with a healthcare professional before making significant dietary adjustments.

39.6 Calcium and Vitamin D for Bone Health during Menopause

Estrogen plays a crucial role in maintaining bone health by inhibiting bone breakdown. As estrogen levels decline during menopause, women become more susceptible to bone loss and osteoporosis. Adequate intake of calcium and vitamin D is essential for preserving bone density and reducing the risk of fractures.

Good dietary sources of calcium include dairy products, leafy greens, tofu, and fortified plant-based milk. Vitamin D can be obtained through sunlight exposure and dietary sources such as fatty fish, egg yolks, and fortified foods.

Supplementation with calcium and vitamin D may be necessary for some women, particularly those with low bone density or limited sun exposure. A healthcare professional can assess individual needs and recommend appropriate supplements.

39.7 The Impact of Exercise on Menopause and Weight

Regular physical activity is beneficial for women during menopause for various

reasons:

- Weight management: Exercise helps maintain a healthy weight and reduce the risk of weight gain during menopause.

- Bone health: Weight-bearing exercises, such as walking, jogging, and strength training, help promote bone density and reduce the risk of osteoporosis.

- Mood and well-being: Physical activity releases endorphins, which can improve mood and reduce stress and anxiety.

- Cardiovascular health: Exercise supports heart health and reduces the risk of cardiovascular disease, which may increase during menopause.

A combination of cardiovascular exercises, strength training, and flexibility exercises is ideal for overall health and well-being during menopause. Engaging in activities that bring joy and satisfaction can also enhance adherence to an exercise routine.

39.8 Foods to Avoid for Menopause Symptom Management

Certain foods and beverages may exacerbate menopause symptoms and should be consumed in moderation:

- Caffeine: Caffeine can trigger hot flashes and may disrupt sleep. Limiting or avoiding caffeinated beverages can help manage these symptoms.

- Spicy foods: Spicy foods may induce hot flashes or worsen existing symptoms in some women. Reducing spicy food intake can be beneficial for symptom management.

- Alcohol: Alcohol can disrupt sleep and may trigger hot flashes in some women. Reducing alcohol consumption can improve sleep quality and overall well-being.

39.9 Mindful Eating for Emotional Well-being during Menopause

Mindful eating is a beneficial practice for women during menopause, especially as emotional eating and food cravings may become more prevalent. Mindful eating involves paying attention to hunger and fullness cues, savoring the taste and texture of food, and eating with intention and awareness.

During times of stress or emotional turmoil, women may turn to food for comfort. Mindful eating can help break this cycle and promote a healthier relationship with food.

Practicing mindfulness during meals can also improve digestion and nutrient absorption. Taking time to chew food thoroughly and eating in a relaxed environment supports optimal digestion.

39.10 Seeking Support and Guidance for Menopause and Weight

Managing menopause and weight changes can be a unique and challenging experience for women. Seeking support and guidance from healthcare professionals, including registered dietitians and menopause specialists, can be invaluable during this stage of life.

A healthcare professional can provide personalized nutrition recommendations, address specific symptoms and concerns, and develop a comprehensive plan for managing menopause-related changes and maintaining a healthy weight.

In conclusion, menopause is a transformative stage in a woman's life that requires attention to nutritional needs and overall well-being. Understanding the impact of menopause on weight, metabolism, and hormonal health is essential for making informed dietary choices. Incorporating phytoestrogen-rich foods, calcium, and vitamin D for bone health, and engaging in regular exercise can support overall health during menopause. Additionally, mindful eating can promote emotional well-being and a positive relationship with food. Seeking support from healthcare professionals can provide tailored guidance for navigating menopause and promoting a healthy weight during this life stage. By embracing a balanced diet and lifestyle, women can experience menopause with grace and vitality.

Chapter 40: Nutrition for Preparing for Surgery and Recovery

Surgery is a significant medical intervention that requires careful preparation and post-operative care. Nutrition plays a crucial role in supporting the body's healing processes, minimizing complications, and promoting a smooth recovery. In this chapter, we will explore the essential aspects of nutrition to consider before and after surgery to optimize surgical outcomes and aid in the recovery process.

40.1 The Impact of Nutrition on Surgical Outcomes

Good nutrition is essential for maintaining overall health and can have a significant impact on surgical outcomes. Proper nutrition before surgery can help optimize the body's ability to withstand the stress of surgery and support the immune system. Adequate nutrition is also critical for wound healing, tissue repair, and infection prevention.

Malnutrition or nutrient deficiencies can impair the body's ability to heal, increase the risk of complications, and delay recovery. Therefore, it is vital for individuals undergoing surgery to pay close attention to their nutritional status and make necessary dietary adjustments.

40.2 Preparing for Surgery: Nutritional Considerations

In the days leading up to surgery, individuals should focus on consuming a balanced diet that provides essential nutrients. A diet rich in fruits, vegetables, whole grains, lean proteins, and healthy fats can support the body's immune function and reduce inflammation.

It is essential to avoid crash diets or drastic changes in eating habits right before surgery, as this can potentially weaken the body and compromise the surgical outcome. Instead, opt for consistent, nourishing meals that provide a steady supply of nutrients.

If surgery is scheduled far in advance, individuals can work with a registered dietitian to develop a personalized nutrition plan that addresses specific dietary needs and health conditions.

40.3 The Importance of Hydration Before and After Surgery

Proper hydration is crucial for supporting the body's functions and optimizing surgical outcomes. Dehydration can impede blood flow, reduce oxygen delivery to tissues, and impair wound healing. Therefore, it is essential to ensure adequate hydration before surgery.

On the day of surgery, individuals should follow their healthcare provider's instructions regarding fasting and drinking clear fluids. After surgery, maintaining proper hydration is equally important to promote healing and prevent complications.

40.4 Nutrition for Wound Healing and Tissue Repair

After surgery, the body enters a phase of wound healing and tissue repair, which requires an increased demand for nutrients. Protein, vitamins, and minerals are especially important during this time.

Protein plays a critical role in tissue repair and wound healing. Adequate protein intake helps the body produce new tissue and collagen, which is essential for wound closure and scar formation.

Vitamins and minerals, such as vitamin C, zinc, and copper, are also vital for wound healing. These nutrients support the formation of collagen and promote a healthy immune response.

40.5 Protein Requirements for Surgery and Recovery

The protein needs of individuals undergoing surgery are typically higher than those of healthy individuals. Protein helps repair damaged tissues, support the immune system, and prevent muscle loss during periods of inactivity.

The recommended protein intake during the recovery period may vary depending on the extent of the surgery and individual factors such as age, weight, and overall health. It is essential for individuals to work with their healthcare providers or a registered dietitian to determine their specific protein requirements.

40.6 Micronutrients and Their Role in Healing

In addition to macronutrients like protein, micronutrients play a crucial role in supporting the healing process. Nutrients such as vitamin A, vitamin C, vitamin E, zinc, and copper are involved in collagen synthesis, antioxidant defense, and immune function.

Fruits and vegetables are excellent sources of essential vitamins and minerals. Including a variety of colorful fruits and vegetables in the diet can help ensure a sufficient intake of these important micronutrients.

40.7 Managing Inflammation and Swelling with Diet

Inflammation and swelling are natural responses to surgery and are part of the body's healing process. However, excessive inflammation can lead to pain and discomfort. Certain foods and nutrients can help manage inflammation and reduce swelling.

Omega-3 fatty acids, found in fatty fish, flaxseeds, and chia seeds, have anti-inflammatory properties. Incorporating these foods into the diet can help modulate the body's inflammatory response.

Additionally, spices such as turmeric and ginger have potent anti-inflammatory effects and can be used in cooking or consumed as herbal teas.

40.8 Post-Surgery Nutrition and Pain Management

After surgery, many individuals experience pain and discomfort, which can affect their appetite and eating habits. However, maintaining proper nutrition during the recovery period is crucial for supporting the healing process.

If pain or discomfort makes it challenging to eat solid foods, opting for softer or pureed foods can be helpful. Additionally, consuming nutrient-dense liquids, such as smoothies or soups, can provide essential nutrients without putting too much strain on the digestive system.

Pain medications may also affect appetite or digestion. It is essential to communicate any concerns about eating or nutrition with healthcare providers, as they can provide guidance and adjustments to pain management strategies if needed.

40.9 Dietary Strategies for a Smooth Recovery

To promote a smooth recovery after surgery, individuals can focus on incorporating specific dietary strategies into their post-operative nutrition plan:

- Eating small,

frequent meals: Eating smaller, more frequent meals can be easier on the digestive system and help maintain steady energy levels.

- Prioritizing nutrient-dense foods: Choosing nutrient-dense foods ensures that the body receives essential vitamins and minerals for healing and recovery.

- Including probiotics: Probiotics can support gut health and immune function during the recovery process. Fermented foods like yogurt, kefir, and sauerkraut are excellent sources of probiotics.

- Avoiding excessive sugar and processed foods: High-sugar and processed foods can promote inflammation and hinder the healing process. It is best to minimize their intake during recovery.

40.10 Working with Healthcare Professionals for Optimal Surgery Nutrition

Before and after surgery, it is essential for individuals to work closely with their healthcare team, including surgeons, registered dietitians, and other medical professionals. They can provide personalized guidance and recommendations based on an individual's specific health needs, surgical procedure, and recovery goals.

In conclusion, proper nutrition is essential for preparing the body for surgery, optimizing surgical outcomes, and supporting the recovery process. Adequate protein, vitamins, minerals, and hydration play a critical role in wound healing, tissue repair, and managing inflammation. By following a balanced and nutrient-rich diet and collaborating with healthcare professionals, individuals can enhance their chances of a successful surgery and a smooth recovery.

Chapter 41: Nutrition for Digestive Health and Weight Loss

Maintaining a healthy digestive system is crucial for overall well-being and can significantly impact weight management. The gut plays a pivotal role in nutrient absorption, metabolism, and the elimination of waste. It is also home to trillions of microorganisms collectively known as the gut microbiome, which influences various aspects of health, including digestion, immune function, and even weight regulation. In this chapter, we will explore the connection between the gut microbiome and weight management, the role of probiotics and prebiotics in gut health and weight loss, the importance of fiber for digestion and weight control, and the impact of the gut-brain axis on appetite and eating behavior.

41.1 The Gut Microbiome and Its Role in Weight Management

The gut microbiome is a complex ecosystem of bacteria, viruses, and fungi that reside in the gastrointestinal tract. It plays a crucial role in breaking down and fermenting certain dietary components that our bodies cannot digest on their own. In turn, these microorganisms produce beneficial byproducts, such as short-chain fatty acids, which have been linked to improved gut health and reduced inflammation.

Recent research has unveiled the role of the gut microbiome in weight management. An imbalance in the gut microbiome, known as dysbiosis, has been associated with weight gain and obesity. Dysbiosis can lead to increased calorie extraction from food and the release of pro-inflammatory molecules that contribute to weight gain.

On the other hand, a diverse and balanced gut microbiome is associated with better weight management and overall health. Consuming a variety of fiber-rich foods, prebiotics, and probiotics can promote the growth of beneficial gut bacteria and support a healthy gut environment.

41.2 Probiotics and Prebiotics for Gut Health and Weight Loss

Probiotics are live bacteria that provide health benefits when consumed in adequate amounts. They can be found in fermented foods such as yogurt, kefir, kimchi, sauerkraut, and kombucha. Probiotics help maintain a balanced gut microbiome by increasing the population of beneficial bacteria and inhibiting the growth of harmful ones.

Several studies have indicated that probiotics may support weight loss efforts. They can modulate gut hormones that influence appetite and satiety, potentially reducing overall food intake. Additionally, probiotics have been linked to improved insulin sensitivity, which can aid in weight management.

Prebiotics, on the other hand, are non-digestible fibers found in certain plant foods, such as garlic, onions, bananas, and asparagus. Prebiotics serve as food for probiotics, helping them thrive and multiply in the gut. By including prebiotic-rich foods in the diet, individuals can support the growth of beneficial gut bacteria, which may positively impact weight management.

41.3 The Impact of Fiber on Digestive Function and Weight

Fiber is a type of carbohydrate found in plant-based foods that is not fully broken down or absorbed by the body. It is essential for digestive health as it adds bulk to stools, facilitates regular bowel movements, and prevents constipation. Beyond its digestive benefits, fiber also plays a critical role in weight management.

High-fiber foods are often low in calories and can help create a feeling of fullness, reducing overall calorie intake. Additionally, soluble fiber can form a gel-like substance in the digestive tract, which slows down the digestion and absorption of nutrients, including carbohydrates and sugars. This can help stabilize blood sugar levels and reduce spikes in insulin, promoting weight loss and reducing the risk of insulin resistance.

Incorporating a variety of fiber-rich foods into the diet, such as fruits, vegetables, whole grains, legumes, and nuts, can be beneficial for digestive health and weight management.

41.4 Fermented Foods for Improved Gut Health and Metabolism

Fermented foods undergo a process of lacto-fermentation, where natural bacteria feed on the sugars and starches in the food, creating lactic acid. This process preserves the food and enhances its flavor while also providing probiotics and beneficial enzymes.

Consuming fermented foods can promote a healthy gut microbiome and improve digestive function. The probiotics found in fermented foods help maintain a balanced gut ecosystem, supporting digestion, nutrient absorption, and immune function.

In addition to their digestive benefits, fermented foods may also impact metabolism. Some studies suggest that the probiotics found in fermented foods can influence the way the body stores and processes fats, potentially supporting weight management.

41.5 Gut-Brain Axis and Its Influence on Appetite and Eating Behavior

The gut-brain axis refers to the bidirectional communication between the gut and the brain. The gut microbiome produces various neuroactive compounds, including neurotransmitters and metabolites, that can influence brain function and behavior.

For example, certain gut bacteria can produce neurotransmitters like serotonin, which plays a role in regulating mood and appetite. An imbalance in gut bacteria may impact the production of these neurotransmitters, potentially affecting eating behavior and food cravings.

Additionally, the gut-brain axis can influence the way we respond to stress. Chronic stress can alter the gut microbiome, leading to changes in appetite and eating patterns. Stress eating, or emotional eating, is a common response to stress and can contribute to weight gain.

By nurturing a healthy gut environment through proper nutrition and gut-friendly foods, individuals may support a balanced gut-brain axis, potentially reducing stress-related eating behaviors and promoting healthier food choices.

41.6 Addressing Gut Imbalances to Support Weight Loss

Addressing gut imbalances, such as dysbiosis, is crucial for effective weight management. A

personalized approach that includes dietary changes and lifestyle modifications can help restore a healthy gut environment and promote weight loss.

One of the first steps is to focus on a diverse and nutrient-rich diet. Consuming a variety of whole foods, including fruits, vegetables, whole grains, lean proteins, and healthy fats, can support the growth of beneficial gut bacteria and improve gut health.

Eliminating or reducing the intake of highly processed foods, sugary beverages, and artificial additives can also be beneficial for gut health. These foods can negatively impact gut bacteria and contribute to inflammation and weight gain.

In some cases, healthcare professionals may recommend specific probiotic supplements to restore gut balance. However, it is essential to consult with a qualified healthcare provider or registered dietitian before starting any supplementation.

41.7 Hydration and Its Effect on Digestion and Weight Management

Hydration is essential for proper digestion and nutrient absorption. Water helps move food through the digestive tract, facilitating the breakdown and absorption of nutrients. Insufficient water intake can lead to constipation and hinder digestion.

Drinking adequate water throughout the day can also support weight management. Sometimes, the body may interpret thirst as hunger, leading to unnecessary snacking or overeating. Staying well-hydrated can help differentiate between thirst and hunger cues, potentially reducing overall calorie intake.

For optimal hydration, aim to drink at least eight cups (64 ounces) of water per day, or more if needed, depending on factors such as climate, activity level, and individual needs.

41.8 Foods for Gut Healing and Improved Nutrient Absorption

Certain foods can promote gut healing and improve nutrient absorption, which is essential for overall health and weight management.

Bone broth is a nutrient-rich liquid made by simmering animal bones and connective tissues. It is a rich source of collagen, gelatin, and various minerals. Collagen and gelatin are essential for gut lining repair and can support gut health and digestion.

Foods high in glutamine, an amino acid, are also beneficial for gut healing. Glutamine is used as fuel by the cells lining the digestive tract and supports the repair of damaged gut tissue. Sources of glutamine include poultry, fish, dairy, and certain plant-based foods like beans and spinach.

Furthermore, zinc-rich foods, such as oysters, pumpkin seeds, and beef, can also support gut healing and improve nutrient absorption. Zinc is crucial for maintaining the integrity of the intestinal lining and supporting the gut barrier.

Including these gut-healing foods as part of a balanced diet can enhance gut health, improve nutrient absorption, and support overall well-being.

41.9 The Role of Gut Health in Reducing Inflammation and Weight Gain

Inflammation is a natural immune response to protect the body from injury and infection. However, chronic inflammation can be harmful and is associated with various health conditions, including obesity.

A balanced and diverse gut microbiome can help reduce systemic inflammation. The production of short-chain fatty acids by beneficial gut bacteria has anti-inflammatory properties and can protect against inflammation-related weight gain.

Eating a diet rich in anti-inflammatory foods, such as fatty fish, nuts, seeds, leafy greens, and colorful fruits and vegetables, can support gut health and reduce inflammation.

Additionally, avoiding highly processed and sugary foods can help reduce inflammation and its associated health risks.

41.10 Creating a Gut-Nourishing Diet Plan for Weight Loss

Developing a gut-nourishing diet plan can be a valuable tool for weight management and overall well-being. Consider the following principles when creating a gut-nourishing diet:

1. Emphasize plant-based foods: Fruits, vegetables, whole grains, legumes, nuts, and seeds provide a diverse range of nutrients and support a healthy gut microbiome.

2. Incorporate probiotics and fermented foods: Yogurt, kefir, sauerkraut, kimchi, and kombucha can introduce beneficial probiotics to support gut health.

3. Consume prebiotic-rich foods: Garlic, onions, leeks, asparagus, bananas, and whole grains contain prebiotic fibers that feed beneficial gut bacteria.

4. Opt for fiber-rich choices: Fiber supports digestion, promotes a feeling of fullness, and aids in weight management. Include a variety of fiber-rich foods in your diet.

5. Stay hydrated: Drinking enough water is crucial for digestion, nutrient absorption, and overall gut health.

6. Minimize processed foods: Limiting processed foods and sugary beverages can reduce inflammation and support a healthy gut environment.

7. Listen to your body: Pay attention to how different foods make you feel and adjust your diet accordingly. Everyone's gut is unique, and individual responses to certain foods may vary.

8. Seek professional guidance: If you have specific gut health concerns or digestive issues, consult with a registered dietitian or healthcare provider to develop a personalized nutrition plan.

In conclusion, nutrition plays a critical role in maintaining a healthy gut and supporting weight loss efforts. The gut microbiome and its balance of beneficial bacteria can significantly impact digestion, metabolism, and weight management. By incorporating probiotics, prebiotics, fiber-rich foods, and gut-healing nutrients into the diet, individuals can support gut health and improve weight management. Additionally, creating a gut-nourishing diet plan can help optimize digestion, reduce inflammation, and promote overall well-being. As always, it is essential to work with healthcare professionals or registered dietitians to develop a personalized nutrition plan that meets individual needs and goals.

Chapter 42: Nutrition for Enhancing Exercise Performance and Weight Loss

42.1 Optimal Nutrition for Fueling Physical Activity and Workouts

Nutrition plays a vital role in supporting exercise performance and weight loss efforts. Properly fueling the body before, during, and after workouts can enhance energy levels, optimize performance, and aid in weight management.

To fuel physical activity effectively, individuals should focus on consuming a balanced diet that includes a variety of macronutrients and micronutrients. Carbohydrates are the body's primary source of energy, and they are especially important for endurance exercises. Whole grains, fruits, vegetables, and legumes are excellent sources of complex carbohydrates that provide sustained energy.

Protein is essential for muscle repair and growth, making it crucial for individuals engaging in strength training or resistance exercises. Lean meats, poultry, fish, eggs, dairy products, and plant-based protein sources like tofu and legumes are excellent options for meeting protein needs.

Healthy fats, found in foods like avocados, nuts, seeds, and olive oil, are essential for overall health and can provide a secondary source of energy during prolonged exercise sessions.

Hydration is equally critical for supporting exercise performance. Dehydration can lead to decreased performance, fatigue, and impaired recovery. Before, during, and after workouts, it is essential to drink enough water to maintain proper hydration.

42.2 Pre-Workout Nutrition for Increased Energy and Performance

Pre-workout nutrition aims to provide the body with the necessary nutrients to perform optimally during exercise. The timing and composition of pre-workout meals depend on individual preferences and the intensity and duration of the activity.

A balanced pre-workout meal should include a combination of carbohydrates, protein, and a small amount of healthy fats. Carbohydrates provide readily available energy, while protein helps preserve muscle mass during exercise.

Examples of pre-workout meals include a turkey sandwich on whole-grain bread, a smoothie with fruits and protein powder, or Greek yogurt with berries and granola.

Individuals who prefer to exercise on an empty stomach can have a small snack or a piece of fruit to provide a quick source of energy.

42.3 Carbohydrates for Sustained Endurance and Weight Loss

Carbohydrates play a crucial role in supporting sustained endurance and weight loss. Endurance exercises, such as running, cycling, or swimming, rely heavily on the body's carbohydrate stores for energy.

Consuming carbohydrates before and during prolonged exercises can help maintain energy levels and delay fatigue. This is especially important for individuals engaging in activities lasting longer than one hour.

For weight loss, the timing and type of carbohydrates can also be essential. Choosing complex carbohydrates, such as whole grains, vegetables, and legumes, over refined carbohydrates can help stabilize blood sugar levels and promote a feeling of fullness, reducing the likelihood of overeating after workouts.

42.4 Protein and Its Role in Muscle Repair and Fat Loss

Protein is essential for muscle repair, growth, and maintenance. Engaging in regular exercise, particularly strength training, puts additional stress on the muscles, making adequate protein intake crucial for recovery.

Consuming protein after workouts can help stimulate muscle protein synthesis and enhance recovery. Including a source of protein in post-workout meals or snacks can promote muscle repair and growth.

In addition to supporting muscle health, protein can also play a role in weight loss. Protein-rich foods help increase feelings of fullness and can aid in weight management by reducing overall calorie intake.

For individuals looking to enhance exercise performance and support weight loss, incorporating lean sources of protein, such as chicken, turkey, fish, tofu, beans, and lentils, into their diet can be beneficial.

42.5 Hydration Strategies for Exercise and Weight Management

Staying adequately hydrated is essential for overall health and exercise performance. Proper hydration can help regulate body temperature, improve endurance, and prevent dehydration-related issues like muscle cramps and fatigue.

Before exercise, individuals should aim to drink about 16-20 ounces of water two to three hours before the workout. During exercise, especially during intense or prolonged activities, it is essential to drink water regularly to replace fluids lost through sweat.

For exercise sessions lasting longer than one hour, consuming beverages containing electrolytes can help maintain electrolyte balance and support performance. Sports drinks or electrolyte-infused water can be suitable choices for prolonged workouts.

Hydration is also essential for weight management. Sometimes, the body can confuse thirst with hunger, leading to unnecessary calorie consumption. Drinking enough water throughout the day can help distinguish between thirst and hunger cues, reducing the likelihood of overeating.

42.6 Post-Workout Nutrition for Recovery and Muscle Preservation

Post-workout nutrition is crucial for promoting recovery and muscle preservation. After exercise, the body is primed to absorb nutrients and replenish energy stores.

A balanced post-workout meal should include a combination of carbohydrates and protein. Carbohydrates help replenish glycogen stores, while protein aids in muscle repair and growth.

Timing is essential for post-workout nutrition. Consuming a meal or snack containing carbohydrates and protein within one to two hours after exercise can optimize recovery and support muscle health.

Examples of post-workout meals include grilled chicken with sweet potatoes and vegetables, a quinoa salad with chickpeas and leafy greens, or

a protein smoothie with fruits and Greek yogurt.

42.7 Nutrient Timing for Exercise and Weight Loss Goals

Nutrient timing refers to the strategic timing of meals and snacks to optimize exercise performance and weight loss goals. While nutrient timing can be beneficial, individual preferences and schedules should be considered.

For individuals focusing on weight loss, consuming most of their carbohydrates before and after workouts can help maximize energy during exercise while controlling overall calorie intake.

On the other hand, athletes or individuals aiming to enhance exercise performance may benefit from consuming carbohydrates before and during intense or prolonged workouts to maintain energy levels and support endurance.

42.8 Supplements for Exercise Performance and Weight Management

While proper nutrition from whole foods should always be the primary focus, some individuals may consider using supplements to support exercise performance and weight management.

Popular supplements for exercise performance include creatine, beta-alanine, and branched-chain amino acids (BCAAs). Creatine can improve strength and power, beta-alanine can reduce fatigue during high-intensity exercise, and BCAAs can help prevent muscle breakdown during endurance exercises.

For weight management, some individuals may use supplements like whey protein, green tea extract, or conjugated linoleic acid (CLA) to support their goals.

It is essential to approach supplements with caution and consult with healthcare professionals or registered dietitians before using them. While some supplements can be beneficial, others may not be necessary or may have potential side effects.

42.9 Creating a Customized Nutrition Plan for Active Weight Loss

Creating a customized nutrition plan for active weight loss involves considering individual preferences, activity level, and weight loss goals.

A diet plan that supports weight loss should focus on a slight calorie deficit, achieved by balancing calorie intake from macronutrients (carbohydrates, protein, and fats) with energy expenditure from exercise.

Incorporating whole, nutrient-dense foods into the diet, such as fruits, vegetables, lean proteins, whole grains, and healthy fats, can provide essential nutrients while promoting satiety.

Regular physical activity should be an integral part of the weight loss plan. Combining proper nutrition with exercise can enhance weight loss results and promote overall health and well-being.

42.10 Integrating Exercise and Nutrition for Long-Term Weight Maintenance

Integrating exercise and nutrition for long-term weight maintenance is essential for sustaining weight loss results. Adopting a balanced and sustainable approach to both diet and exercise can lead to better compliance and overall success.

As individuals progress in their weight loss journey, they may need to adjust their nutrition and exercise plan to accommodate changes in their body composition and metabolism.

Consistency is key to long-term success. Finding a balanced and enjoyable exercise routine and adhering to a nutritious diet can lead to lasting weight management and improved overall health.

Working with healthcare professionals or registered dietitians can provide valuable guidance and support in developing a personalized plan for exercise performance and weight loss that aligns with individual needs and goals. A comprehensive approach that includes both nutrition and exercise can set the foundation for a healthier and more active lifestyle, promoting overall well-being and vitality.

Chapter 43: Nutrition for Hormonal Balance and Sustainable Weight Loss

43.1 The Impact of Hormones on Metabolism and Weight Regulation

Hormones play a crucial role in regulating various physiological processes, including metabolism and weight management. Hormonal imbalances can significantly influence how the body processes and stores energy, affecting weight loss and gain.

One of the key hormones involved in metabolism and weight regulation is insulin. Insulin is released by the pancreas in response to elevated blood sugar levels after consuming carbohydrates. Its primary function is to facilitate the uptake of glucose into cells for energy production or storage. However, chronically elevated insulin levels can lead to insulin resistance, impairing the body's ability to use stored fat for energy, thus promoting weight gain.

Other hormones, such as cortisol, estrogen, progesterone, and testosterone, also play a role in weight management. For instance, cortisol, known as the stress hormone, can lead to increased fat storage, particularly around the abdominal area, when released excessively due to chronic stress. Estrogen and progesterone fluctuations in women during the menstrual cycle can affect appetite, food cravings, and energy expenditure. Testosterone, although more prominent in males, also influences body composition and muscle mass, affecting overall metabolism.

43.2 Balancing Insulin and Blood Sugar for Weight Management

Maintaining balanced blood sugar levels and insulin sensitivity is crucial for sustainable weight loss. Unstable blood sugar levels can lead to increased hunger, cravings, and overeating, making it challenging to manage weight effectively.

To promote balanced blood sugar levels, individuals should focus on consuming complex carbohydrates, such as whole grains, legumes, and vegetables, which release glucose more slowly into the bloodstream. This helps prevent sudden spikes and crashes in blood sugar levels, reducing the likelihood of overeating.

Pairing carbohydrates with protein and healthy fats can further stabilize blood sugar levels and promote satiety. Including foods like lean proteins, avocados, nuts, and olive oil in meals can slow down the absorption of glucose and help maintain energy levels throughout the day.

Regular physical activity can also improve insulin sensitivity, making the body more efficient at using glucose for energy rather than storing it as fat.

43.3 Hormones and Their Effect on Appetite and Cravings

Hormones play a significant role in regulating appetite and food cravings. Ghrelin, known as the "hunger hormone," increases appetite and signals the brain when it's time to eat. Leptin, on the other hand, is the "satiety hormone" and signals the brain when the body is full and no longer needs to eat.

Hormonal imbalances, such as elevated ghrelin levels or reduced leptin sensitivity, can lead to increased hunger and a higher likelihood of overeating. This can be particularly challenging for individuals trying to lose weight.

In addition to ghrelin and leptin, other hormones, such as serotonin and dopamine, also influence food cravings and eating behavior. Serotonin, often called the "feel-good hormone," is associated with mood and emotional well-being. Low serotonin levels can lead to increased cravings for carbohydrates and sugary foods as a way to temporarily boost mood.

Managing stress and emotional well-being is essential for balancing hormones that affect appetite and cravings. Practices such as mindfulness, meditation, and stress-reduction techniques can help regulate hormones and reduce emotional eating.

43.4 Nutrition Strategies for Supporting Thyroid Function and Weight Loss

The thyroid gland plays a critical role in regulating metabolism and energy expenditure. An underactive thyroid, known as hypothyroidism, can slow down metabolism and lead to weight gain, fatigue, and other health issues.

Supporting thyroid function through proper nutrition is essential for individuals with thyroid imbalances. Iodine is a crucial nutrient for thyroid health, as it is a component of thyroid hormones. Foods rich in iodine include seaweed, iodized salt, and fish.

Selenium is another essential mineral that supports thyroid function. Brazil nuts, tuna, and sardines are excellent sources of selenium.

Including foods rich in zinc, such as oysters, beef, and pumpkin seeds, can also be beneficial for thyroid health.

Consuming a well-balanced diet that provides all essential nutrients is essential for overall hormonal balance and weight management. Prioritizing nutrient-dense foods and avoiding nutrient deficiencies can support thyroid function and metabolic health.

43.5 Addressing Cortisol Imbalance for Stress-Related Weight Gain

Cortisol, the primary stress hormone, plays a vital role in the body's response to stress. In acute situations, cortisol helps the body mobilize energy and cope with stressors. However, chronic stress can lead to persistently elevated cortisol levels, which can contribute to weight gain, particularly around the abdominal area.

When cortisol levels are elevated for prolonged periods, the body may start to store more fat, especially visceral fat, which is linked to an increased risk of metabolic disorders and chronic diseases.

To manage cortisol levels and reduce stress-related weight gain, individuals can adopt stress-reduction techniques such as mindfulness, meditation, yoga, and regular physical activity. Engaging in activities that promote relaxation can help lower cortisol levels and support hormonal balance.

43.6 The Role of Estrogen and Progesterone in Female Weight Management

Hormones such as estrogen and progesterone significantly influence female weight management. Throughout the menstrual cycle, estrogen levels fluctuate, impacting energy expenditure, appetite, and metabolism.

During the follicular phase, which occurs in the first half of the menstrual cycle, estrogen levels gradually increase. This phase is associated with increased insulin sensitivity, which means the body can use carbohydrates more efficiently for energy.

In contrast, during the luteal phase, which occurs in the second half of the menstrual cycle, both estrogen and progesterone levels rise. This phase is associated with increased hunger and food cravings, particularly for sweet and high-calorie foods.

Understanding these hormonal fluctuations can help women adapt their nutrition and exercise strategies throughout their menstrual cycle. During the luteal phase, individuals may benefit from focusing on nutrient-dense foods, managing cravings mindfully, and incorporating regular physical activity.

43.7 Testosterone and Its Influence on Body Composition and Fat Loss

Testosterone is primarily known as a male sex hormone, but it also plays a role in body composition and fat loss for both men and women. Testosterone supports the maintenance and growth of lean muscle mass, which can increase metabolic rate and aid in fat loss.

Men generally have higher testosterone levels than women, which contributes to their higher lean body mass and overall higher metabolic rate. However, women also produce testosterone, albeit in smaller amounts.

Resistance training, such as weightlifting, can help both men and women optimize testosterone levels and support lean muscle mass development. Adequate protein intake is crucial for muscle synthesis, making it an essential nutrient for individuals aiming to improve body composition and promote fat loss.

43.8 Nourishing Adrenal Health for Balanced Hormones and Weight Loss

The adrenal glands, located on top of the kidneys, produce hormones such as cortisol and adrenaline. Chronic stress can lead to adrenal fatigue or dysfunction, impacting overall hormonal balance and contributing to weight gain.

Nourishing adrenal health involves adopting stress-management techniques, ensuring adequate sleep and rest, and consuming a balanced diet rich in nutrients.

Eating a variety of nutrient-dense foods, such as fruits, vegetables, whole grains, lean proteins, and healthy fats, provides essential vitamins and minerals necessary for adrenal function and hormonal balance.

43.9 Nutrition for Supporting Hormonal Health and Sustainable Fat Loss

A balanced and nutritious diet is crucial for supporting hormonal health and sustainable fat loss. Key dietary principles include:

1. Prioritizing Whole Foods: Choosing whole, nutrient-dense foods over processed and sugary options provides essential vitamins, minerals, and antioxidants that support hormonal health.

2. Adequate Protein Intake: Protein is essential for muscle maintenance and repair, which can enhance metabolism and support fat loss. Including lean sources of protein, such as poultry, fish, tofu, and legumes, in meals and snacks is recommended.

3. Healthy Fats: Incorporating healthy fats from sources like avocados, nuts, seeds, and olive oil can support hormone production and aid in satiety.

4. Hydration: Staying hydrated is essential for overall health and hormonal balance. Drinking enough water can support metabolism, digestion, and cellular function.

5. Mindful Eating: Practicing mindful eating can help individuals recognize hunger and fullness cues, manage stress-related eating, and reduce emotional eating.

6. Limiting Processed Foods and Added Sugars: Processed foods and added sugars can contribute to hormonal imbalances and weight gain. Minimizing their intake supports overall health and weight management.

43.10 Seeking Professional Guidance for Hormonal Balance and Weight Management

Hormonal imbalances can be complex and require personalized strategies for effective management. Individuals experiencing significant hormonal issues or struggling with weight management despite healthy lifestyle habits should seek professional guidance.

Registered dietitians, endocrinologists, or other healthcare professionals with expertise in hormonal health can conduct comprehensive assessments, develop personalized plans, and provide ongoing support to promote hormonal balance and sustainable weight loss.

In conclusion, nutrition plays a vital role in hormonal balance and weight management. Balancing insulin, addressing cortisol imbalances, supporting thyroid function, and understanding the impact of hormones on appetite and cravings are essential components of sustainable weight loss. By adopting a balanced and nutrient-dense diet, engaging in regular physical activity, managing stress, and seeking professional guidance when needed, individuals can optimize hormonal health and achieve their weight loss goals in a safe and effective manner.

Chapter 44: Nutrition for Boosting Metabolism and Accelerating Weight Loss

44.1 Understanding Metabolism and Its Impact on Weight Loss

Metabolism refers to the complex set of chemical reactions that occur within the body to convert food into energy. It plays a crucial role in determining the number of calories the body burns at rest (resting metabolic rate or RMR) and during physical activity. Understanding how metabolism works is essential for individuals seeking to accelerate weight loss.

A faster metabolism means the body burns more calories, even at rest, which can support weight loss efforts. However, metabolism is influenced by various factors, including age, genetics, body composition, and hormone levels. As individuals age, their metabolism may naturally slow down, making weight loss more challenging.

While some factors affecting metabolism cannot be changed, lifestyle and dietary choices can play a significant role in optimizing metabolism for weight loss.

44.2 Strategies for Increasing Resting Metabolic Rate (RMR)

Resting metabolic rate (RMR) represents the number of calories the body burns at rest to maintain essential bodily functions, such as breathing, circulation, and cellular processes. Increasing RMR can help individuals burn more calories throughout the day, supporting weight loss.

Several strategies can help boost RMR:

1. Regular Physical Activity: Engaging in regular exercise, such as aerobic activities, strength training, and high-intensity interval training (HIIT), can increase RMR and contribute to weight loss.

2. Building Lean Muscle Mass: Muscle tissue burns more calories than fat tissue, even at rest. Incorporating strength training into the exercise routine can help build lean muscle, contributing to higher RMR.

3. Eating Sufficient Protein: Protein has a higher thermic effect than carbohydrates or fats, meaning the body burns more calories to digest and process it. Including adequate protein in meals can support RMR.

4. Ensuring Adequate Sleep: Sleep is essential for metabolic health. Poor sleep quality and insufficient sleep can negatively impact metabolism and hinder weight loss efforts.

44.3 The Role of High-Intensity Interval Training (HIIT) in Metabolism

High-Intensity Interval Training (HIIT) involves alternating short bursts of intense exercise with periods of rest or lower-intensity exercise. HIIT has gained popularity for its effectiveness in boosting metabolism and supporting weight loss.

HIIT workouts challenge the body and elevate heart rate, promoting excess post-exercise oxygen consumption (EPOC). EPOC refers to the increased caloric expenditure that occurs after exercise as the body works to recover and return to its pre-exercise state. This post-workout caloric burn can contribute to overall weight loss.

In addition to its impact on metabolism, HIIT has been shown to improve cardiovascular health, increase aerobic capacity, and promote fat loss while preserving lean muscle mass.

44.4 The Impact of Strength Training on Basal Metabolic Rate (BMR)

Strength training, also known as resistance training, involves working against resistance to build muscle strength and endurance.

Besides its benefits for muscle development, strength training can significantly impact basal metabolic rate (BMR).

BMR represents the number of calories the body requires to maintain basic physiological functions when at rest. As mentioned earlier, muscle tissue has a higher metabolic rate than fat tissue, meaning individuals with a higher proportion of lean muscle mass tend to have a higher BMR.

Engaging in regular strength training exercises can help individuals build and maintain muscle mass, which can increase BMR. This can lead to higher caloric expenditure at rest and support weight loss goals.

44.5 Thermogenic Foods and Their Effect on Caloric Expenditure

Thermogenic foods, also known as "metabolism-boosting" foods, have been suggested to increase the body's caloric expenditure during digestion and processing. These foods often contain compounds or nutrients that can temporarily raise body temperature and stimulate metabolism.

Common thermogenic foods include:

1. Spicy Foods: Certain compounds found in chili peppers, such as capsaicin, can increase metabolism and promote fat oxidation.

2. Green Tea: Green tea contains catechins and caffeine, which have been shown to have a thermogenic effect, boosting metabolism and promoting fat loss.

3. Coffee: Coffee contains caffeine, which can temporarily increase metabolic rate and energy expenditure.

4. Ginger: Ginger has thermogenic properties that may stimulate metabolism and support digestion.

While thermogenic foods can have a modest impact on metabolism, they are not a substitute for overall healthy eating and lifestyle habits. Incorporating these foods as part of a balanced diet can complement weight loss efforts.

44.6 Metabolism-Boosting Nutrients and Their Food Sources

Certain nutrients play a role in supporting metabolism and weight loss. Including these nutrients in the diet can help optimize metabolic function:

1. Protein: Adequate protein intake can increase the thermic effect of food, supporting caloric expenditure during digestion and promoting muscle preservation during weight loss. Good sources of protein include lean meats, fish, poultry, tofu, legumes, and dairy products.

2. Iron: Iron is essential for transporting oxygen in the blood and supporting metabolic function. Sources of iron include red meat, poultry, beans, lentils, spinach, and fortified cereals.

3. B Vitamins

: B vitamins, including B6, B12, and folate, play a role in energy metabolism and the breakdown of carbohydrates, proteins, and fats. Foods rich in B vitamins include whole grains, leafy greens, meats, eggs, and nuts.

4. Iodine: Iodine is crucial for thyroid hormone production, which regulates metabolism. Iodine-rich foods include iodized salt, seaweed, fish, and dairy products.

5. Magnesium: Magnesium is involved in over 300 biochemical reactions in the body, including energy production and muscle function. Sources of magnesium include leafy greens, nuts, seeds, whole grains, and legumes.

44.7 Meal Frequency and Its Influence on Metabolic Rate

The frequency of meals and snacks throughout the day can influence metabolic rate and energy expenditure. Some studies suggest that frequent, smaller meals may boost metabolism, while others show little difference between meal frequencies.

It's important to note that individual responses to meal frequency can vary. Some people may feel better with more frequent, smaller meals, while others prefer fewer, larger meals.

Ultimately, focusing on overall calorie intake, nutrient balance, and food quality is more important than meal frequency for weight loss and metabolic health. Eating meals that are satisfying, nutrient-dense, and appropriate in portion size can support a healthy metabolism.

44.8 Hydration and Its Connection to Metabolism and Weight Loss

Staying adequately hydrated is essential for overall health and can also impact metabolism and weight loss. Water is involved in numerous bodily processes, including metabolism and energy expenditure.

Drinking enough water can temporarily increase resting metabolic rate (RMR) and the thermic effect of food (TEF), leading to a slight boost in caloric expenditure. Additionally, staying hydrated can support optimal digestion, nutrient absorption, and waste elimination.

Hydrating with water or low-calorie beverages throughout the day is recommended for those aiming to support a healthy metabolism and promote weight loss.

44.9 Managing Stress and Sleep for a Healthy Metabolism

Chronic stress and poor sleep can negatively impact metabolism and hinder weight loss efforts. High levels of stress can lead to increased cortisol production, which may contribute to weight gain, especially around the abdominal area.

Additionally, inadequate sleep can disrupt hormonal balance and affect appetite-regulating hormones, leading to increased hunger and potential overeating.

Managing stress through relaxation techniques, exercise, and engaging in activities that bring joy can support a healthy metabolism. Prioritizing sleep and establishing a consistent sleep schedule can also optimize metabolic function and support weight loss goals.

44.10 Implementing Metabolism-Enhancing Nutrition Strategies for Weight Loss

Incorporating metabolism-enhancing nutrition strategies into a well-balanced diet and lifestyle can support weight loss efforts. Here are some tips for optimizing metabolism:

1. Include Protein in Every Meal: Adequate protein intake can support muscle preservation, increase the thermic effect of food, and boost metabolism.

2. Engage in Regular Exercise: Both aerobic exercises, such as walking, running, and swimming, and strength training can increase metabolism and contribute to weight loss.

3. Stay Hydrated: Drinking enough water throughout the day can temporarily boost metabolic rate and support digestion.

4. Prioritize Sleep: Aim for 7-9 hours of quality sleep each night to support hormonal balance and metabolic health.

5. Manage Stress: Engage in stress-reducing activities, such as yoga, meditation, or spending time in nature, to support a healthy metabolism.

6. Avoid Extreme Diets: Crash diets and extreme calorie restriction can slow down metabolism and lead to nutrient deficiencies. Focus on balanced, nutrient-dense eating for sustainable weight loss.

7. Limit Processed Foods and Sugars: Processed foods and added sugars can negatively impact metabolism and contribute to weight gain. Opt for whole, unprocessed foods instead.

8. Consult with a Professional: For personalized guidance and support, consider consulting with a registered dietitian or healthcare professional with expertise in weight management and metabolism.

In conclusion, optimizing metabolism is essential for individuals aiming to accelerate weight loss. By understanding the factors that influence metabolic rate and implementing metabolism-boosting nutrition strategies, individuals can support their weight loss goals in a safe and effective manner. Combining these strategies with regular physical activity, adequate sleep, and stress management can create a comprehensive approach to weight loss and overall well-being.

Chapter 45: Nutrition for Sustainable Weight Loss Maintenance

45.1 The Importance of Transitioning from Weight Loss to Maintenance

Achieving weight loss is a significant accomplishment, but the journey does not end there. Transitioning from weight loss to weight maintenance is a crucial step in ensuring long-term success and preventing weight regain. Sustainable weight loss maintenance involves adopting new habits, making lifestyle changes, and developing a positive relationship with food and oneself.

It's essential to understand that maintaining weight loss requires as much effort and dedication as the weight loss phase. During this transition, individuals need to focus on building healthy habits that support their new weight and promote overall well-being.

45.2 Understanding Metabolic Adaptation and Its Impact on Maintenance

Metabolic adaptation refers to the body's natural response to weight loss. As individuals lose weight, their metabolism may slow down, and their caloric needs may decrease. This adaptation is the body's way of preserving energy and preventing further weight loss.

During the maintenance phase, individuals should be aware of metabolic adaptation and adjust their caloric intake accordingly. It's essential to find the right balance of calories to support weight maintenance without regaining lost weight.

45.3 Finding Your Maintenance Caloric Intake and Nutrient Balance

Determining the appropriate caloric intake for weight maintenance requires a balance of factors, including age, gender, activity level, and metabolic rate. Various online calculators and formulas can provide estimates, but consulting with a registered dietitian or nutritionist can offer personalized guidance.

In addition to caloric intake, the nutrient balance is essential for maintaining health and preventing nutrient deficiencies. A well-rounded diet that includes a variety of nutrient-dense foods is crucial for long-term weight maintenance.

45.4 Building Sustainable Eating Habits for Long-Term Success

Sustainable eating habits are the foundation of successful weight maintenance. Crash diets and extreme restrictions are not sustainable in the long run and can lead to weight regain. Instead, individuals should focus on creating a balanced and flexible eating plan that they can maintain for life.

Practicing mindful eating, enjoying meals without distractions, and listening to hunger and fullness cues can promote healthy eating habits. Avoiding emotional eating and finding alternative ways to cope with stress and emotions are also vital for long-term success.

45.5 Incorporating Regular Physical Activity into Your Lifestyle

Physical activity plays a significant role in weight maintenance. Regular exercise not only supports weight management but also improves overall health and well-being. Find an exercise routine that you enjoy and can sustain over time.

Combining cardiovascular exercises with strength training can help preserve muscle mass and boost metabolism. Aim for at least 150 minutes of moderate-intensity aerobic activity or 75 minutes of vigorous-intensity aerobic activity per week, along with muscle-strengthening activities on two or more days per week.

45.6 Mindful Eating and Portion Control for Weight Maintenance

Practicing mindful eating during the maintenance phase can help individuals stay in tune with their body's needs and prevent overeating. Mindful eating involves being present during meals, savoring each bite, and recognizing hunger and fullness cues.

Portion control is also essential for weight maintenance. Even healthy foods can contribute to weight gain if consumed in excessive amounts. Measuring portions, using smaller plates, and avoiding eating straight from the package can help with portion control.

45.7 Celebrating Non-Scale Victories and Nourishing Self-Compassion

Weight maintenance is not just about the number on the scale. Celebrate non-scale victories, such as increased energy, improved fitness levels, and better mood. Acknowledge the progress made in building healthy habits and staying committed to a healthy lifestyle.

Nourishing self-compassion is essential during the maintenance phase. Be kind to yourself, recognize that everyone has ups and downs, and focus on progress rather than perfection. If there are occasional setbacks, use them as learning experiences and continue moving forward.

45.8 Monitoring Progress and Adjusting Nutritional Intake as Needed

Regularly monitoring progress is essential for weight maintenance. Keep track of food intake, physical activity, and any changes in weight or body measurements. This can help identify any patterns or areas that need adjustment.

If weight starts to creep up, consider reassessing caloric intake and activity levels. Make gradual adjustments to bring the body back into balance. Avoid drastic changes, as they may lead to an unsustainable cycle of restriction and overindulgence.

45.9 Creating a Supportive Environment for Weight Maintenance

A supportive environment can significantly impact weight maintenance success. Surround yourself with positive influences, such as friends, family, or support groups, who understand your goals and encourage healthy habits.

Avoid environments or situations that trigger unhealthy eating behaviors or negative self-talk. Surround yourself with people who uplift and support your efforts to maintain a healthy weight and lifestyle.

45.10 Embracing a Balanced and Enjoyable Lifestyle for Lasting Results

Weight maintenance is not about rigid rules or extreme measures. Embrace a balanced and enjoyable lifestyle that includes a variety of nutritious foods, regular physical activity, and stress-reducing practices.

Find joy in cooking and experimenting with new recipes that align with your nutritional goals. Remember that a healthy lifestyle is a lifelong journey, and finding pleasure in the process will contribute to sustainable weight maintenance.

In conclusion, transitioning from weight loss to weight maintenance requires a shift in mindset and a commitment to long-term health and well-being. Understanding metabolic adaptation, finding the right caloric intake, and building sustainable habits are essential for maintaining weight loss. By incorporating regular physical activity, practicing mindful eating, and creating a supportive environment, individuals can embrace a balanced and enjoyable lifestyle that leads to lasting results. Seeking professional guidance and support, when needed, can also be beneficial in navigating the challenges and triumphs of weight maintenance. Remember that every individual's journey is unique, and finding what works best for you is key to sustainable weight loss maintenance.

Chapter 46: Nutrition for Enhancing Mental Clarity and Focus

In today's fast-paced world, maintaining mental clarity and focus is essential for productivity, performance, and overall well-being. The foods we eat play a significant role in supporting cognitive function and brain health. Proper nutrition can enhance memory, concentration, and mental alertness while reducing the risk of age-related cognitive decline. In this chapter, we will explore the impact of nutrition on cognitive function and discuss specific brain-boosting nutrients and dietary strategies to enhance mental clarity and focus.

46.1 The Impact of Nutrition on Cognitive Function

The brain is a highly metabolically active organ that requires a constant supply of energy and nutrients to function optimally. Nutrients from the foods we eat provide the building blocks for neurotransmitters, the chemical messengers that facilitate communication between brain cells. Therefore, nutrition plays a critical role in supporting cognitive function and brain health.

A well-balanced diet that includes a variety of nutrient-dense foods can help enhance memory, attention, and overall cognitive performance. On the other hand, a poor diet characterized by excessive intake of processed foods, sugary beverages, and unhealthy fats may lead to cognitive impairment and increase the risk of neurodegenerative diseases.

46.2 Brain-Boosting Nutrients: Omega-3 Fatty Acids and Antioxidants

Omega-3 fatty acids, particularly docosahexaenoic acid (DHA), are crucial for brain health. DHA is a major component of cell membranes in the brain and is involved in the formation of synapses, which are vital for learning and memory. Foods rich in omega-3 fatty acids include fatty fish (e.g., salmon, mackerel, and sardines), chia seeds, flaxseeds, and walnuts.

Antioxidants, such as vitamins C and E, as well as polyphenols, play a crucial role in protecting the brain from oxidative stress and inflammation. These compounds can help preserve cognitive function and reduce the risk of cognitive decline. Foods rich in antioxidants include colorful fruits and vegetables, nuts, seeds, and green tea.

46.3 Hydration and Its Influence on Cognitive Performance

Proper hydration is essential for maintaining mental clarity and focus. Dehydration can lead to cognitive impairments, including reduced attention, memory, and problem-solving skills. Drinking an adequate amount of water throughout the day can help support optimal cognitive function.

In addition to water, certain beverages like green tea can offer brain-boosting benefits due to their antioxidant content and the presence of compounds that may improve cognitive function.

46.4 Foods that Support Memory and Concentration

Several foods are known for their memory-enhancing properties and their ability to support concentration. For example, berries, especially blueberries, are rich in antioxidants and flavonoids that can improve memory and cognitive function. Dark chocolate, in moderation, contains flavonoids that may enhance blood flow to the brain and boost memory.

Leafy green vegetables, such as spinach and kale, are rich in vitamins and minerals that support brain health. Nuts and seeds, particularly almonds and pumpkin seeds, are excellent sources of vitamin E, an antioxidant that may help protect brain cells from oxidative damage.

46.5 Nutritional Strategies for Improved Mental Alertness

To improve mental alertness, it is essential to stabilize blood sugar levels through balanced meals and snacks. Avoiding large fluctuations in blood sugar can help maintain steady energy levels and mental focus throughout the day.

Incorporating protein-rich foods like lean meats, fish, eggs, and legumes into meals can help provide sustained energy and support cognitive function. Including complex carbohydrates from whole grains, fruits, and vegetables can also help maintain steady blood sugar levels.

46.6 The Role of Gut Health in Cognitive Function

The gut-brain axis is a bidirectional communication system between the gut and the brain that plays a significant role in cognitive function and mental health. The gut is home to trillions of microbes that influence various aspects of brain health, including mood, memory, and cognition.

Consuming a diet rich in prebiotic foods (e.g., garlic, onions, and bananas) and probiotic foods (e.g., yogurt, kefir, and sauerkraut) can support a healthy gut microbiome, positively impacting cognitive function.

46.7 Managing Stress and Its Effect on Brain Function

Chronic stress can have detrimental effects on cognitive function and memory. High levels of stress hormones, such as cortisol, can impair memory retrieval and reduce attention span.

Practicing stress-reducing techniques such as meditation, deep breathing, and spending time in nature can help mitigate the negative effects of stress on the brain.

46.8 The Connection Between Sleep and Mental Clarity

Adequate sleep is crucial for cognitive function, memory consolidation, and overall brain health. During sleep, the brain undergoes important processes that promote learning, memory formation, and cellular repair.

Prioritizing restful sleep and maintaining a consistent sleep schedule can significantly enhance mental clarity and focus.

46.9 Nutrition for Mental Health and Emotional Well-Being

The foods we eat can also influence our mood and emotional well-being. Diets high in processed foods and unhealthy fats have been associated with an increased risk of depression and anxiety.

On the other hand, consuming a nutrient-dense diet that includes whole grains, lean proteins, healthy fats, fruits, and vegetables can support mental health and emotional well-being.

46.10 Building a Brain-Boosting Diet Plan for Enhanced Focus and Productivity

To build a brain-boosting diet plan, consider incorporating the following foods and dietary strategies:

1. Omega-3 Fatty Acids: Include fatty fish, chia seeds, flaxseeds, and walnuts in your diet to support brain health.

2. Antioxidants: Consume a variety of colorful fruits and vegetables, nuts, seeds, and green tea to provide your brain with important antioxidants.

3. Hydration: Stay adequately hydrated by drinking water throughout the day to support cognitive function.

4. Memory-Enhancing Foods: Include berries, dark chocolate (in moderation), leafy greens, and nuts and seeds to enhance memory and concentration.

5. Balanced Meals: Opt for balanced meals that include a combination of lean proteins, complex carbohydrates, and healthy fats to stabilize blood sugar levels and support mental alertness.

6. Gut-Healthy Foods: Incorporate prebiotic and probiotic-rich foods to support a healthy gut microbiome, which positively impacts cognitive function.

7. Stress Management: Practice stress-reducing techniques such as meditation, deep breathing, and spending time in nature to mitigate the negative effects of stress on the brain.

8. Sleep: Prioritize restful sleep and maintain a consistent sleep schedule to support cognitive function and memory consolidation.

Conclusion

Nutrition plays a crucial role in enhancing mental clarity and focus. Brain-boosting nutrients such as omega-3 fatty acids and antioxidants, along with proper hydration and gut-healthy foods, can support cognitive function and brain health. Managing stress, prioritizing sleep, and adopting a nutrient-dense diet can also contribute to improved mental alertness and productivity.

By building a brain-boosting diet plan and making lifestyle choices that support cognitive function, individuals can enhance their focus, memory, and overall brain health for optimal performance in all aspects of life. Remember that small dietary and lifestyle changes can have a significant impact on mental clarity and well-being, making it essential to prioritize nutrition for brain health and cognitive   function.

Chapter 47: Nutrition for a Healthy Immune System and Weight Management

47.1 The Link Between Nutrition and Immune Health

The immune system is a complex network of cells, tissues, and organs that work together to defend the body against harmful pathogens and maintain overall health. Proper nutrition plays a crucial role in supporting immune function and promoting a healthy immune response. Nutrient deficiencies can weaken the immune system, making the body more susceptible to infections and illnesses.

A well-balanced diet that includes a variety of vitamins, minerals, antioxidants, and other essential nutrients is essential for optimal immune function. Additionally, maintaining a healthy weight is closely linked to immune health, as obesity can impair immune responses and increase the risk of chronic diseases.

47.2 The Role of Nutrients in Supporting Immune Function

Several nutrients play a vital role in supporting immune function:

- Vitamin C: Known for its immune-boosting properties, vitamin C helps stimulate the production and function of immune cells. Citrus fruits, berries, bell peppers, and leafy greens are excellent sources of vitamin C.

- Vitamin D: This vitamin is essential for regulating immune responses and promoting immune cell function. Exposure to sunlight and consuming fatty fish, fortified dairy products, and egg yolks can help maintain adequate vitamin D levels.

- Zinc: Zinc is involved in the production and activation of immune cells. Foods rich in zinc include lean meats, poultry, beans, nuts, and seeds.

- Vitamin A: Critical for maintaining the integrity of the skin and mucosal surfaces, vitamin A helps create a barrier against pathogens. Sweet potatoes, carrots, spinach, and liver are good sources of vitamin A.

- Vitamin E: An antioxidant that helps protect immune cells from oxidative damage. Nuts, seeds, and vegetable oils are rich sources of vitamin E.

47.3 The Gut-Immune Connection and Its Impact on Weight

The gut and the immune system are closely interconnected. The gut houses a large portion of the body's immune cells and plays a vital role in immune responses. Additionally, the gut microbiome, the community of microorganisms residing in the gut, has a profound impact on immune function.

A balanced gut microbiome is crucial for maintaining immune homeostasis and preventing chronic inflammation. The gut microbiome also plays a role in weight management. Imbalances in the gut microbiome, such as dysbiosis, have been linked to weight gain and obesity. Conversely, a healthy and diverse gut microbiome is associated with better weight management.

47.4 Foods that Enhance Immune Responses and Aid Weight Loss

Certain foods have immune-enhancing properties and can support weight loss efforts:

- Berries: Rich in antioxidants and phytochemicals, berries help reduce inflammation and boost immune function. They are also low in calories and can be included in a weight loss diet.

- Cruciferous Vegetables: Broccoli, cauliflower, and Brussels sprouts are rich in vitamins, minerals, and fiber, supporting both immune health and weight management.

- Fatty Fish: Fatty fish like salmon and mackerel are excellent sources of omega-3 fatty acids, which have anti-inflammatory effects and support immune function.

- Lean Proteins: Chicken, turkey, fish, and plant-based proteins like legumes and tofu provide essential amino acids for immune cell function while supporting weight loss by promoting satiety.

- Green Tea: Rich in antioxidants, green tea supports immune health and may aid weight loss by boosting metabolism.

47.5 The Importance of Antioxidants for Immune Support

Antioxidants play a crucial role in immune support by neutralizing harmful free radicals and reducing oxidative stress. Free radicals are unstable molecules that can damage cells and tissues, leading to inflammation and impaired immune responses. Antioxidants help protect immune cells from oxidative damage, ensuring their proper function.

In addition to vitamin C and vitamin E, other antioxidants like selenium, beta-carotene, and flavonoids also contribute to immune support. Including a wide variety of colorful fruits and vegetables in the diet can provide a diverse range of antioxidants.

47.6 Probiotics and Prebiotics for a Balanced Immune System

Probiotics are beneficial live bacteria that can support a healthy gut microbiome. They help maintain a balanced gut flora and support immune function. Fermented foods like yogurt, kefir, sauerkraut, and kimchi are rich sources of probiotics.

Prebiotics, on the other hand, are non-digestible fibers that promote the growth of beneficial gut bacteria. Foods like garlic, onions, bananas, and asparagus are good sources of prebiotics.

A healthy gut microbiome not only enhances immune function but also supports weight management by influencing metabolism and nutrient absorption.

47.7 Hydration and Its Influence on Immune Health and Metabolism

Proper hydration is essential for overall health, including immune function and metabolism. Water is necessary for the proper functioning of immune cells and helps transport nutrients throughout the body. Dehydration can impair immune responses and lead to fatigue, which may impact physical activity and weight management efforts.

Staying well-hydrated can also support weight loss by promoting feelings of fullness and enhancing the body's ability to metabolize stored fat.

47.8 The Impact of Sleep and Stress on Immunity and Weight Management

Quality sleep is crucial for immune function and weight management. During sleep, the body undergoes important processes that support immune responses and tissue repair. Chronic sleep deprivation can weaken the immune system and increase the risk of infections.

Stress also plays a significant role in immune function and weight management. Chronic stress can lead to inflammation and immune dysfunction, making the body more susceptible to illnesses

. Moreover, stress can trigger emotional eating and disrupt healthy eating patterns, leading to weight gain.

47.9 Lifestyle Habits for a Resilient Immune System and Sustainable Weight Loss

In addition to proper nutrition, certain lifestyle habits can support a resilient immune system and sustainable weight loss:

- Regular Exercise: Physical activity can enhance immune function, promote weight loss, and reduce the risk of chronic diseases.

- Stress Management: Practicing stress-reducing techniques such as mindfulness, meditation, and yoga can support immune health and weight management.

- Sufficient Sleep: Prioritize getting 7-9 hours of quality sleep each night to support immune function and aid weight management efforts.

- Avoid Smoking and Excessive Alcohol: Smoking and excessive alcohol consumption can weaken the immune system and hinder weight loss efforts.

47.10 Prioritizing Immune Health for Successful Long-Term Weight Management

Prioritizing immune health through proper nutrition, hydration, sleep, and stress management is essential for successful long-term weight management. A strong immune system can help protect the body from infections and illnesses, ensuring that individuals can stay active and maintain their weight loss goals.

Integrating immune-boosting foods, antioxidants, probiotics, and prebiotics into a well-balanced diet can optimize immune function while supporting weight loss efforts. Additionally, adopting a healthy lifestyle that includes regular exercise, stress reduction, and sufficient sleep can further strengthen the immune system and contribute to successful weight management in the long run.

By recognizing the interplay between nutrition, immune health, and weight management, individuals can make informed choices to achieve overall well-being and maintain a healthy weight throughout their lives. Seeking guidance from healthcare professionals and registered dietitians can provide personalized recommendations and support for optimizing immune health and achieving sustainable weight loss.

Chapter 48: Nutrition for Enhanced Sleep and Weight Loss

48.1 The Impact of Nutrition on Sleep Quality

Nutrition plays a significant role in influencing sleep quality. The foods we eat can affect the production of certain neurotransmitters and hormones that regulate sleep-wake cycles. Additionally, the timing of meals and the types of nutrients consumed can impact sleep patterns and overall sleep quality.

One of the key hormones involved in sleep regulation is melatonin. Melatonin is responsible for signaling the body when it's time to sleep and promoting restful sleep. Foods rich in tryptophan, an amino acid that serves as a precursor to melatonin, can support the production of this sleep-inducing hormone. Tryptophan-rich foods include turkey, chicken, nuts, seeds, and dairy products.

On the other hand, consuming large, heavy meals close to bedtime can disrupt sleep as the body diverts its energy toward digestion instead of promoting relaxation and rest. Spicy or acidic foods, caffeine, and alcohol can also interfere with sleep patterns and should be avoided in the evening.

48.2 Foods that Promote Restful Sleep and Weight Loss

Certain foods contain nutrients that promote restful sleep while also supporting weight loss efforts:

- Cherries: Cherries are a natural source of melatonin, which can help regulate sleep-wake cycles and improve sleep quality.

- Almonds: Almonds are rich in magnesium, a mineral that helps relax muscles and promote calmness, making it easier to fall asleep.

- Kiwi: Kiwi is another fruit that contains compounds that may improve sleep quality and duration.

- Herbal Teas: Herbal teas like chamomile, valerian root, and passionflower have soothing properties that can promote relaxation and improve sleep.

- Fatty Fish: Fatty fish like salmon and tuna are rich in omega-3 fatty acids, which have been associated with improved sleep quality.

48.3 The Connection Between Sleep and Hormones Regulating Appetite

Sleep has a direct impact on the hormones that regulate appetite and satiety. Leptin and ghrelin are two key hormones involved in hunger regulation. Leptin is responsible for signaling fullness and suppressing appetite, while ghrelin stimulates hunger and increases food intake.

Lack of sleep or poor sleep quality can disrupt the balance of these hormones. Sleep deprivation is associated with decreased leptin levels and increased ghrelin levels, leading to an increase in appetite and food cravings. This disruption in hunger hormones can lead to overeating and weight gain over time.

48.4 Hydration and Its Influence on Sleep and Weight Management

Proper hydration is essential for overall health, including sleep quality and weight management. Dehydration can lead to discomfort and restless sleep. Drinking enough water throughout the day can help improve sleep quality and support weight loss efforts.

However, it's essential to balance hydration during the evening to avoid disruptions to sleep caused by frequent trips to the bathroom. It's a good practice to moderate fluid intake closer to bedtime while ensuring adequate hydration throughout the day.

48.5 The Role of Micronutrients in Sleep Regulation and Metabolism

Micronutrients, such as vitamins and minerals, also play a role in sleep regulation and metabolism. Magnesium, for example, is involved in more than 600 enzymatic reactions in the body, including those that support relaxation and sleep. Adequate magnesium intake has been linked to better sleep quality.

Vitamins B6 and B12 are also important for sleep regulation, as they are involved in the synthesis of neurotransmitters that influence sleep and mood.

48.6 Creating a Sleep-Supportive Evening Routine

Establishing a sleep-supportive evening routine can significantly improve sleep quality and support weight loss efforts. Some practices that can be incorporated into an evening routine include:

- Setting a consistent bedtime: Going to bed and waking up at the same time each day helps regulate the body's internal clock and improve sleep quality.

- Limiting screen time: Exposure to the blue light emitted by screens (phones, computers, TVs) in the evening can interfere with the production of melatonin and disrupt sleep. It's best to limit screen time at least an hour before bedtime.

- Relaxation techniques: Practicing relaxation techniques such as deep breathing, meditation, or gentle stretching can help calm the mind and body, making it easier to fall asleep.

- Creating a comfortable sleep environment: Ensure the bedroom is conducive to sleep by keeping it cool, dark, and quiet.

48.7 Sleep Environment and Its Effect on Sleep Quality and Weight

The sleep environment plays a crucial role in sleep quality and weight management. A comfortable and supportive mattress and pillow can improve sleep posture and reduce discomfort, contributing to better sleep quality.

Furthermore, a clutter-free and peaceful sleep environment can promote relaxation and help reduce stress, which can positively impact sleep and support weight management efforts.

48.8 Managing Stress and Its Impact on Sleep and Weight Loss

Stress is a common factor that can interfere with both sleep and weight management. Chronic stress can lead to sleep disturbances, such as difficulty falling asleep or staying asleep.

Moreover, stress triggers the release of cortisol, a hormone that can promote weight gain, particularly in the abdominal area. Managing stress through relaxation techniques, exercise, and mindfulness practices can improve sleep quality and support weight loss goals.

48.9 The Importance of Exercise in Improving Sleep and Weight Management

Regular exercise is beneficial for both sleep quality and weight management. Physical activity can help reduce stress and anxiety, leading to better sleep.

Moreover, exercise promotes the release of endorphins, the body's natural feel-good

chemicals, which can contribute to improved mood and better sleep quality.

Engaging in regular exercise can also support weight management by increasing calorie expenditure and promoting fat loss while preserving lean muscle mass.

48.10 Integrating Nutrition and Sleep for Overall Well-being and Sustainable Weight Loss

Integrating nutrition and sleep into a comprehensive approach to overall well-being is essential for sustainable weight loss and optimal health.

By adopting a balanced diet that includes sleep-supportive nutrients, managing stress, and establishing healthy sleep habits, individuals can enhance sleep quality and support their weight loss journey effectively.

Moreover, addressing sleep-related issues and improving sleep quality can positively impact hormonal regulation, appetite control, and emotional well-being, all of which play a significant role in sustainable weight loss.

Seeking guidance from healthcare professionals or registered dietitians can provide personalized recommendations and support in creating a nutrition and sleep plan tailored to individual needs and goals.

Chapter 49: Nutrition for a Healthy Liver and Weight Management

49.1 The Role of the Liver in Detoxification and Metabolism

The liver is one of the most vital organs in the body and plays a central role in various metabolic processes, including detoxification. It is responsible for filtering and processing toxins, drugs, and metabolic waste, ensuring they are safely eliminated from the body. Additionally, the liver plays a critical role in metabolism, including the breakdown and storage of carbohydrates, fats, and proteins.

A healthy liver is essential for overall well-being, including weight management. When the liver is functioning optimally, it can efficiently metabolize nutrients, regulate blood sugar levels, and aid in fat metabolism.

49.2 Foods that Support Liver Health and Aid Weight Loss

Certain foods can support liver health and contribute to weight loss efforts:

- Leafy Greens: Leafy greens such as spinach, kale, and arugula are rich in antioxidants and phytochemicals that support liver function.

- Cruciferous Vegetables: Vegetables like broccoli, cauliflower, and Brussels sprouts contain compounds that enhance liver detoxification.

- Citrus Fruits: Citrus fruits like oranges, lemons, and grapefruits are high in vitamin C, which supports liver health.

- Turmeric: The active compound in turmeric, curcumin, has potent anti-inflammatory and antioxidant properties that benefit liver function.

- Green Tea: Green tea contains catechins, which have been shown to protect the liver from damage and support weight loss.

- Nuts and Seeds: Nuts and seeds provide healthy fats, antioxidants, and nutrients that benefit liver health.

49.3 Hydration and Its Influence on Liver Function and Weight Management

Adequate hydration is crucial for liver function and weight management. Water helps flush out toxins and waste products from the liver, promoting optimal detoxification processes. Staying hydrated also supports digestion and nutrient absorption, which are essential for overall health and weight management.

Moreover, proper hydration can aid in weight loss by promoting satiety and reducing the likelihood of overeating. Sometimes, thirst can be mistaken for hunger, leading to unnecessary calorie consumption. Drinking enough water throughout the day can help prevent this and support weight loss goals.

49.4 The Impact of Nutrient-Dense Foods on Liver Health

A diet rich in nutrient-dense foods provides essential vitamins, minerals, and antioxidants that promote liver health. These nutrients play a vital role in supporting liver function and protecting against oxidative stress and inflammation.

Consuming a variety of colorful fruits and vegetables, whole grains, lean proteins, and healthy fats can provide the liver with the necessary nutrients it needs to function optimally. Additionally, nutrient-dense foods are generally lower in calories, making them an excellent choice for those looking to manage their weight while nourishing their liver.

49.5 Managing Inflammation and Fatty Liver with Nutrition

Inflammation in the liver can lead to various liver conditions, including non-alcoholic fatty liver disease (NAFLD). NAFLD is characterized by the accumulation of fat in the liver cells, which can impair liver function and lead to more severe liver issues if left untreated.

To manage inflammation and promote a healthy liver, it's essential to focus on an anti-inflammatory diet. This diet includes foods rich in omega-3 fatty acids, such as fatty fish and flaxseeds, as well as foods high in antioxidants, like berries and leafy greens.

49.6 The Role of Antioxidants in Liver Protection and Weight Loss

Antioxidants are compounds that help neutralize harmful free radicals in the body, reducing oxidative stress and inflammation. The liver can be susceptible to oxidative damage, especially when exposed to toxins or an unhealthy diet.

A diet rich in antioxidants from fruits, vegetables, and other whole foods can help protect the liver from damage and support its detoxification processes. By reducing inflammation and supporting liver health, antioxidants can also contribute to weight loss efforts, as inflammation can interfere with the body's ability to burn fat effectively.

49.7 Foods to Avoid for Liver Health and Weight Management

To support a healthy liver and effective weight management, it's essential to avoid or limit certain foods that can be detrimental to liver function:

- Sugary and Processed Foods: Excessive consumption of sugary and processed foods can lead to insulin resistance and increase the risk of fatty liver disease.

- Trans Fats: Trans fats, often found in fried and processed foods, are harmful to the liver and can contribute to weight gain.

- Alcohol: Alcohol is a known toxin to the liver and can lead to liver inflammation and damage. It is crucial to moderate or avoid alcohol for optimal liver health.

- High-Sodium Foods: Foods high in sodium can contribute to water retention and bloating, putting extra strain on the liver and cardiovascular system.

- Excessive Caffeine: While moderate caffeine consumption is generally safe for most people, excessive caffeine intake can strain the liver and interfere with sleep, which is important for weight management.

49.8 Exercise and Its Effect on Liver Function and Weight Loss

In addition to nutrition, regular physical activity is crucial for both liver health and weight management. Exercise helps improve blood flow to the liver, supporting its detoxification processes and overall function.

Physical activity also aids in weight loss by increasing calorie expenditure and promoting fat loss while preserving lean muscle mass. Combined with a balanced diet, exercise can contribute to sustainable weight management and improved liver health.

49.9 Lifestyle Habits for a Healthy Liver and Sustainable Weight Management

In addition to nutrition and exercise, certain lifestyle habits can promote a healthy liver and support sustainable weight management:

- Manage Stress:

Chronic stress can negatively impact the liver and contribute to weight gain. Engaging in stress-reducing activities such as meditation, yoga, or spending time in nature can be beneficial.

- Get Quality Sleep: Prioritize getting enough sleep each night, as poor sleep can impair liver function and hinder weight loss efforts.

- Avoid Smoking: Smoking is harmful to the liver and overall health. Quitting smoking can have significant benefits for liver health and weight management.

- Limit Medications: Some medications can be hard on the liver. If possible, work with a healthcare professional to reduce the number of medications taken and explore natural alternatives.

49.10 Nurturing a Liver-Friendly Diet for Overall Wellness and Weight Loss

In conclusion, a liver-friendly diet is not only essential for liver health but also for sustainable weight management. By incorporating foods that support liver function, managing inflammation, and providing essential nutrients, individuals can enhance their overall wellness and achieve their weight loss goals.

It is important to remember that sustainable weight loss and overall health are the results of a balanced and holistic approach, including a nutrient-rich diet, regular physical activity, stress management, and adequate sleep. By adopting these lifestyle changes and seeking guidance from healthcare professionals or registered dietitians, individuals can optimize their liver health, promote weight loss, and improve their overall well-being.

Chapter 50: The Power of Mindful Eating for Weight Management

50.1 Understanding Mindful Eating and Its Benefits

Mindful eating is an approach to eating that involves paying full attention to the eating experience, including the taste, texture, and aroma of food, as well as the sensations and feelings associated with eating. It is about being present in the moment during meals and developing a deeper connection with the food we consume.

In today's fast-paced world, many people eat mindlessly, consuming food quickly and without much thought. This can lead to overeating, emotional eating, and poor food choices, contributing to weight gain and overall health issues. Mindful eating, on the other hand, encourages individuals to slow down, savor each bite, and listen to their body's hunger and fullness cues.

The benefits of mindful eating extend beyond weight management. It can also lead to improved digestion, reduced stress, and a greater appreciation for food and the act of eating. By cultivating mindfulness in eating habits, individuals can develop a healthier relationship with food and make more conscious choices that support their overall well-being.

50.2 The Impact of Mindfulness on Eating Habits and Weight Loss

Mindfulness has a profound impact on eating habits and weight loss. By practicing mindful eating, individuals become more attuned to their body's signals, distinguishing between physical hunger and emotional hunger. This awareness helps prevent overeating due to emotional triggers, stress, or boredom.

Mindful eating also promotes a greater sense of satiety and satisfaction with meals. When individuals are present and fully engaged in the eating experience, they are more likely to recognize when they are comfortably full, leading to reduced calorie intake and better portion control.

Research has shown that mindfulness-based eating practices can lead to significant improvements in weight management, including reduced binge eating, emotional eating, and cravings for unhealthy foods.

50.3 Mindful Eating Techniques for Curbing Overeating and Emotional Eating

Several techniques can be applied to practice mindful eating and curb overeating and emotional eating:

- Slow Down: Take your time to eat and chew each bite thoroughly. Eating slowly allows your body to register fullness and prevents overeating.

- Remove Distractions: Avoid eating while watching TV, working on the computer, or scrolling through your phone. Focus solely on your meal and the act of eating.

- Engage Your Senses: Pay attention to the taste, texture, and smell of your food. Fully savor each bite and appreciate the flavors.

- Pause Before Eating: Before reaching for a snack or meal, take a moment to check in with your emotions and physical hunger. Are you truly hungry, or are you eating out of boredom or stress?

- Practice Mindful Breathing: Take a few deep breaths before and during meals to center yourself and remain present.

50.4 Building Awareness of Hunger and Fullness Cues for Balanced Eating

One of the essential aspects of mindful eating is building awareness of hunger and fullness cues. By tuning in to these signals, individuals can foster a healthier relationship with food and better manage their weight.

To build awareness of hunger cues:

- Rate Your Hunger: Before eating, rate your hunger on a scale from 1 to 10, with 1 being extremely hungry and 10 being overly full. Aim to start eating when you are at a comfortable level of hunger, around a 3 or 4 on the scale.

- Identify True Hunger: True hunger is a physical sensation in the stomach, often described as a gnawing or empty feeling. Emotional hunger, on the other hand, arises from stress, boredom, or other non-physical triggers. Mindful eating helps individuals differentiate between the two.

To build awareness of fullness cues:

- Check-In During Meals: Pause during meals to assess your level of fullness. Are you still hungry, satisfied, or overly full? Adjust your eating accordingly based on these cues.

- Listen to Your Body: Practice listening to your body and stopping when you feel satisfied, even if there is food left on your plate.

50.5 Mindfulness-Based Stress Reduction for Weight Management

Stress can have a significant impact on eating habits and weight management. Many individuals turn to food for comfort or stress relief, leading to emotional eating and weight gain. Mindfulness-based stress reduction (MBSR) techniques can help break this cycle and promote healthier coping mechanisms.

MBSR involves practicing mindfulness meditation and yoga to cultivate awareness of the present moment and reduce stress. By incorporating mindfulness practices into daily life, individuals can better manage stress and minimize the impact it has on their eating behaviors.

When stress is managed effectively, emotional eating is less likely to occur, and individuals can make more conscious choices regarding food intake. This can lead to more balanced eating habits and support weight management goals.

50.6 Mindful Meal Planning and Preparation for Weight Loss

Mindful eating isn't just about what happens during meals; it starts with thoughtful meal planning and preparation. By applying mindfulness to meal planning, individuals can make intentional choices that align with their health and weight management goals.

When planning meals mindfully:

- Consider Nutrient Density: Choose nutrient

-dense foods that provide essential vitamins, minerals, and other nutrients without excess calories. Opt for a variety of colorful fruits and vegetables, lean proteins, whole grains, and healthy fats.

- Include Balanced Meals: Aim to create balanced meals that incorporate all macronutrients (carbohydrates, proteins, and fats) and provide sustained energy throughout the day.

- Listen to Your Body: Plan meals based on your body's hunger and fullness cues. Avoid skipping meals or eating when not hungry.

50.7 Incorporating Mindful Eating in Social and Dining Out Situations

Practicing mindful eating doesn't have to be limited to eating at home. It can also be applied in social settings and while dining out:

- Be Mindful of Portions: Be mindful of portion sizes, especially when served large portions at restaurants. Consider sharing a meal with a friend or taking leftovers home.

- Engage in Conversation: Engaging in conversation during meals can help slow down eating and prevent overeating. Focus on connecting with others rather than solely on the food.

- Choose Mindfully: When dining out, choose foods mindfully, considering both taste preferences and nutritional value.

50.8 The Connection Between Mindfulness and Satiety

Mindfulness and satiety are closely connected. By being present and fully engaged in the eating experience, individuals can enhance their sense of satiety during meals.

Satiety is the feeling of fullness and satisfaction that occurs after eating. Mindful eating helps individuals recognize these signals, preventing overeating and promoting a feeling of contentment with smaller portions.

The act of slowing down and savoring each bite allows the brain and body to register the food's nourishment fully. As a result, individuals are less likely to feel the need to continue eating beyond their actual hunger level.

50.9 Using Mindful Eating to Break Unhealthy Eating Patterns

Mindful eating can be a powerful tool for breaking unhealthy eating patterns and habits. It helps individuals become more aware of emotional triggers and the reasons behind their food choices.

By identifying emotional eating triggers, individuals can find alternative ways to cope with stress, boredom, or other emotional states. Mindful eating can also help break the cycle of restrictive eating followed by overindulgence, leading to a more balanced approach to food and sustainable weight management.

50.10 Embracing a Mindful and Intuitive Approach to Eating for Sustainable Weight Management

Embracing a mindful and intuitive approach to eating is key to sustainable weight management and overall well-being. This approach involves:

- Listening to Your Body: Pay attention to your body's hunger and fullness cues and honor them.

- Practicing Self-Compassion: Be kind to yourself and avoid judgment when it comes to food choices and eating behaviors.

- Enjoying Food: Savor the flavors and pleasure of eating without guilt or deprivation.

- Making Conscious Choices: Be mindful of the foods you choose to nourish your body, considering both nutritional value and personal preferences.

- Being Present: Slow down and be fully present during meals, avoiding distractions and multitasking.

- Staying Attuned: Continuously check in with yourself and your body to stay attuned to your needs and make adjustments as necessary.

By adopting mindful and intuitive eating practices, individuals can develop a healthier relationship with food, manage their weight more effectively, and cultivate a greater sense of well-being and balance in their lives. It is essential to remember that mindful eating is a skill that takes time and practice to develop fully. Patience, self-compassion, and a commitment to being present in the eating experience can lead to profound and lasting changes in weight management and overall health.